Biohealth

Biohealth

Beyond Medicalization: Imposing Health

RAYMOND DOWNING

Foreword by WILLIAM RAY ARNEY

PICKWICK *Publications* • Eugene, Oregon

Pickwick Publications
An Imprint of Wipf and Stock Publishers
199 W. 8th Ave., Suite 3
Eugene, OR 97401

www.wipfandstock.com

ISBN 13: 978-1-60899-795-4

Cataloging-in-Publication data:

Downing, Raymond.

    Biohealth : beyond medicalization: imposing health / Raymond Downing ;
foreword by William Ray Arney.

    p. ; cm. — Includes bibliographical references and index(es).

    ISBN 13: 978-1-60899-795-4

    1. Medical innovations—Social aspects—United States. 2. Biotechnology—
Social aspects—United States. 3. Bioethical issues. 4. Biopolitics—United
States. I. Arney, William Ray. II. Title.

RA418.5.M4 D69 2011

Manufactured in the U.S.A.

To Professor Barasa Khwa Otsyula and all of the Family Medicine registrars and graduates in Kenya. As biohealth oozes into Africa, they keep struggling to develop a sane and appropriate African Family Medicine.

And to Jan
Sine qua non

Contents

Foreword

GOOD THINKING AND THE opportunity to live well depend on fine but good distinctions. Raymond Downing uses a historical scalpel to tease out the difference between "biomedicine" and "biohealth." It's a difference that could make a big difference for everyone who comes under the sway of a modern health care system.

Downing's biomedicine is more familiarly known as scientific medicine or clinical medicine, the sort of medical care that took shape in late eighteenth-century Europe under the emerging bio-mechanical conception of the body. Biomedicine is a pretty good good because it works. By the early part of the twentieth century, safer surgical technique and a slowly growing satchel-full of vaccines and drugs helped people avoid or recover from otherwise fatal or disabling diseases and conditions. Biomedicine's goal was to defeat disease and death and in this it acted as a single-combat warrior on behalf of everyone else. Given its fixation on disease and death, biomedicine was not terribly concerned with the arc of its patients' lives. The patient, to biomedicine, was less a person in need of care and human concern and more a vehicle for bringing diseases to the clinic where problems could sometimes be fixed. Doctors knew their work was bound to the field described by a disease and limited to periods of illness.

"The Patient as a Person" made its first appearance in medical textbooks in 1950; that was the title of the first chapter of Tinsley Harrison's then-new book, *Principles of Internal Medicine.* Thinking of patients as people, subject to all human vicissitudes, set the stage for the development of biohealth. Downing argues that the good of biomedicine became, by 1980, completely overshadowed by biohealth, which is, he says, a corruption of biomedicine. Under biohealth's map for becoming a perpetual presence in people's lives, medicine turns away from defeating disease and death and turns toward the management of living. Chronic disease brought some people under life-long medical surveillance. Screening insisted that non-sick people come into the clinic in search of signs of diseases that are possible but not yet diagnosed. The concept of risk changed possible but not-yet diseases into conditions that are only more or less probable, threats from beyond the horizon. Under the aegis of risk, the modern physician is relieved of definitively answering the screened person who reasonably wants to know, "Am I sick?"; the physician can retreat behind a cloud of statistics and say something like, "You have a significantly elevated chance of becoming sick in the future." And finally, an ethos of personal responsibility, especially responsibility for one's "lifestyle," creates in people a life-long anxiety that urges them toward joining the team for managing their own living. Biohealth invites people to carry the ghost of the clinic with them throughout their lives. Biohealth offers people "optimal life course trajectories" in exchange for constant attentiveness. Attentiveness to what? According to biohealth, life occurs in a bio-psycho-social-eco system, so the answer is that one must be attentive to everything.

But this books shows that the regime of biohealth demands attentiveness to everything except that which matters. Downing reveals the demonic underside of biohealth when he says, "Biohealth skillfully directs our attention away from the fundamental causes of ill health—disparities in wealth, trade imbalances, and the rest—and tells us as individuals or communities that it's up to us. It is an understandable strategy . . . Biohealth is . . . part of the technological system, a system that is not interested in addressing disparities in wealth, trade imbalances, and so on because it is the system that creates them." Biomedicine succeeded if it fixed bodily injuries and insults; biohealth succeeds if it finally conceals the root causes of our dis-eased world. In the end, from his position as a Western-trained physician working in Africa, he invokes a notion of "African healing wisdom" in which "the health of an individual could not be separated from the health of a community." Instead of pursuing a "healthy lifestyle," Downing reminds us of older wisdom traditions that corporately valued community-based well-being and human flourishing.

What difference can knowing this difference between biomedicine and biohealth make to those of us in the technologically advanced West?

Ivan Illich, one of Downing's intellectual heroes, once said, "The certainty that you can do without is one of the most efficacious ways of convincing yourself, no matter where you stand on the intellectual or emotional ladder, that you are free." He imagined that people might renounce biohealth and all it has to offer—conscientiously, thoughtfully, deliberately do without it—so we might become more aware both of what ails us and of the sources of well-being and human flourishing articulated in tradition and manifest in well-founded communities everywhere. Biohealth invites anxious attentiveness to all that is on evidence-based medicine's menu of threats and risks. Illich offered a different invitation. He wrote, "I invite all to shift their gaze, their thoughts, from worrying about health care to cultivating the art of living. And today, with equal importance, to the art of suffering, the art of dying." Downing seems to be saying, let us stop worrying about how to manage our lives and begin again to imagine how best to bear and, thereby, enjoy the living that is the gift of our creation.

—William Ray Arney
Friday Harbor, Washington

Preface

Hospitals: The Corruption of Hospitality

HOSPITALITY IS AN ANCIENT and semi-sacred duty in virtually all cultures.[1] When Odysseus returned home, Athena gave him a beggar's disguise, meaning his subjects could not recognize him. Nevertheless, a swineherd welcomed him. His rationale: "rudeness to a stranger is not decency, poor though he may be. . . . All wanderers and beggars come from Zeus." In the tale of the Trojan War, Paris violated Helen's hospitality, and her husband Menelaus killed him. The subsequent victory over Troy was seen as divine vengeance on abused hospitality.

Both dynamics—hospitality and its abuse—are evident in the Jewish story of Abraham and Lot. Abraham lavishly welcomed three strangers to his house, strangers who then predicted that ninety-year-old Sarah would become pregnant. The same strangers went on to visit Lot in Sodom, and he also welcomed them. However, several young men came to Lot's house intent on abusing the visitors. The very next day Sodom was destroyed by fire and brimstone. To what extent was this a judgment on a culture that loses respect for hospitality? This Jewish theme of hospitality continued into the Christian era: the early church was admonished not to neglect showing hospitality to strangers, "for thereby some have entertained angels unawares" (Hebrews 13:2 KJV).

Many contemporary cultures assume the same obligations for hospitality. In the African understanding, hospitality is one of the chief

1. This review is primarily based on Ivan Illich's paper "Hospitality and Pain." Other sources include the Bible; Claiborne, *Roots of English,* 114; Magesa, *African Religion.* 62–65; and personal correspondence from Bill Arney to help elucidate Illich's analysis of the Good Samaritan.

virtues, and its opposite, greed, is one of the most grievous wrongs. But hospitality in Africa is far more than "being nice"; its purpose is to enhance life itself in all its dimensions. "Hospitality is a form of worship" says one African proverb. Hospitality builds community—and in Africa, without community, there is no humanity. Another African proverb says "Life is when you are together, alone you are an animal."

Hospitality, then, has been a nearly universal obligation. However, the beginning of the Christian Era in Europe brought a new twist to the story. While Jews had accepted the duty to show hospitality, they knew that they themselves had been wanderers in need of hospitality; on a spiritual level, they saw themselves as "sojourners on earth" (Psalm 119:19 RSV). Early Christians followed in the same tradition (Hebrews 11:13); in their story of hospitality, the one giving hospitality was a Good Samaritan *who was traveling*. For the Christians in the first few centuries who were politically persecuted and spiritually homeless, their duty to give hospitality could sometimes only be met by giving of themselves, as the Samaritan did. Hospitality became an even deeper obligation— and yet it remained a choice as it was for the Good Samaritan, a radical choice to show hospitality outside of ethnic and political boundaries.

By the early fourth century, that deeper obligation/choice took on a new form. As the Church developed into an institution, and as persecution receded under Constantine, the Church under the authority of the bishops began to offer hospitality for beggars, travelers, and poor people in specific places, *xenodocheia,* on behalf of the entire community. These were unique institutions so far unknown in the Western World, and remarkably successful. When, half a century after Constantine, the apostate Emperor Julian attempted to return the Empire to its pre-Christian deities, he did encourage that they maintain the Christian practice of the *xenodocheia.* This "charity toward strangers," he said, "most contributed to the success" of Christianity. *Xenodocheo* in Greek means hospitality; the *xenodocheia* were the first hospitals.

Now look a bit deeper at the *xenodocheia.* This unique development, noted and praised by an emperor opposed to those who created it, laid the foundation for institutional hospitality—including modern hospitals. Yet ironically it was a corruption of the original intent of that hospitality: the personal choice of each person to give of themselves to those in need. This choice stemmed from a radical freedom to choose whom one will care for and love, undermining the known ethical duty to care primarily for those of one's own kind. This radical new freedom became corrupted first by becoming reduced to only a duty, and then by becoming institutionalized. Institutionalizing hospitality made the "service" much more widely available, and in doing so relieved individuals of the opportunity for that radical freedom to choose to care. This development ignored the deeper truth that practicing hospitality is as important for those who practice it as it is for those who receive it; that it is in fact more blessed to give than to receive. More than this: when those needing hospitality are ill, part of the healing comes from the relationship with those offering the hospitality. Modern hospitals leave very little room for this healing hospitality.

In the last several years of his life, Ivan Illich kept returning to the theme of the old Latin phrase *corruptio optimi quae est pessima*—the corruption of the best is the worst. He saw many of the ills in our modern institutions as resulting from a corruption of something that had been good. In medieval times, the most important developments in the institutional care of sick people opened the door to corruptions of the very goals they set out to accomplish.

This book tells one such modern story. The contemporary scientific power (called biomedicine) to reliably cure many human diseases, and radically change the course of so many others is, if not "the best," certainly very good. But that good has been corrupted—a process parallel to and reprising the replacement of individual hospitality by *xenodocheia*. Biomedicine is very effective in manipulating the mechanisms of disease, making it difficult to criticize. Yet, precisely because of its success, it has today redefined and expanded its mandate of cure, and in the process has redefined health. It has subtly grown beyond what it has rightfully been praised for, moving into areas of our lives previously felt to be the realms of religion, law, culture, and aesthetics. Because of this expansion, biomedicine has become corrupted.

That systemic corruption does not invalidate the good that biomedicine can offer any more than *xenodocheia* invalidates the radical choice of the Good Samaritan to individually care for someone outside his ethnicity—or the benefit of that charity toward strangers that Julian noted. But we must be aware of what happens when biomedicine, like hospitality, becomes corrupted. The result is a way of thinking that becomes a system: a mixture of the original good with its corruption. In order to make clear in this book the difference, I am calling the scientific power of medicine *biomedicine,* and the mixture of that with its corruption *biohealth.* Shortly we will look at the origin of this word.

Acknowledgments

THIS BOOK WAS BORN when I wrote, as an afterthought, chapter 3 of *Death and Life in America*. Appreciation to all who played a part with ideas, opportunity, support, research, or reviewing: Amazon.com, Jan Armstrong, Bill Arney, the Brown-Moi link, Jacques Ellul, Tom Gates, Kristopher Hartwig, Ivan Illich, the Internet, Moi University, and Wipf and Stock Publishers.

1

Biohealth: Introduction

MEDICALIZATION IS THE PROCESS by which more and more areas of our lives come under the authority of medicine. One reason (among many) that this happens is that medicine has something new to offer for yet another of our human dis-eases. But despite these offerings, modern biomedicine does not enjoy unmitigated praise, and criticisms are strongest where biomedicine is most advanced. Because of its reliance on powerful technology, we find biomedicine impersonal, and we find its power dangerous when things go wrong. We aren't sure we want to be subject to that power, especially at the end of life when that power prolongs suffering even while it prolongs life. Many people flee the power of biomedicine and seek alternative and "complementary" modes of healing—only to return when organs fail or bodies are broken. And we must confront how expensive it all is, with progressively smaller benefits for correspondingly larger investments.

The picture is not equally bleak everywhere. Because some places have not yet experienced the best medicine can offer, they also have been spared its excesses; in other places there are systems in place to control the excesses. Nevertheless, many of the criticisms of medicine noted above inevitably follow the expansion of medicine—an expansion that not only offers more for ancient diseases, but is most ready to bring more of the troubles of our lives into the category of disease. Medicalization—both the expanding of what we do for diseases, and the broadened scope of what we call disease—is an inexorable process.

In fact, it is precisely this expansion of medicine that accounts for the criticisms noted above: the increasingly depersonalized technology, the increasing dangers, the increasing cost. What we don't seem to have realized, however, is that these excesses cannot be curbed by education or legislation, because medicalized expansion is inherent in biomedicine. But more than this, medicalization is in some senses complete: we have, potentially at least, brought everything under the authority of medicine. We are now in a phase beyond medicalization,[1] when even health—the "opposite" of medicine's focus, disease—has become medicalized. Biomedicine, assuming it knows what health is, imposes that understanding on everyone. Medicine used to claim authority over the cracks and interruptions in life; now it claims authority over all of life. This is the corruption of biomedicine I am calling biohealth.

The origins of this word are revealing:

Biology was the first "bio-" word in English, with origins at the beginning of the nineteenth century in Europe.[2] It's meaning, from the Greek, is straightforward: *bio* meant life, and *logy* was theory or science, expressed in words (*logos*). By the nineteenth century, it was becoming clear what the differences were between specific substances that were said to be alive (trees, animals) and substances that weren't (rocks, water, air). "Bio" became the prefix that defined this difference. Based on that understanding of life—which by the middle of the nineteenth century was called "protoplasm"—other disciplines such as biochemistry and biophysics came into being. By the very end of the century the word biosphere appeared—a useful term for the relatively new discipline of ecology.

Early in the twentieth century bioelectric and bioluminescent phenomena were described, and the new disciplines of biomechanics and biomathematics were born. This too is when the word biomedical was first used: medicine based on the application of the findings of the biological sciences rather than, say, theories of the humors, or fate, or faith. By the middle of the century the term biotechnology first appeared and brought with it bioengineering and biostatistics.

However, the real explosion in bio- words began in the 1960s and has continued apace since then. The 1960s gave us bionics (an overlap of

1. A less negative view of this phase is Rose, "Beyond Medicalisation," 700–702.

2. Dating of these "bio-" words is from the Merriam-Webster 11th Collegiate Dictionary (2004). Words were often coined earlier than the dictionary dates that reflect when they were accepted as "official" words. Newer unofficial words, biohealth among them, are not in many dictionaries, but are encountered in any internet search engine.

biology and electronics), biorhythm, biodegradable, and bioactive, but also biohazard and biowarfare. In the 1970s we were studying biofeedback and developing biofuels such as biogas, we proposed the holistic biopsychosocial model of health care, and by then we needed the discipline of bioethics. From the 1980s onward we had biopesticides and biopharmaceuticals—and in more academic discussions, biopower and bioplitics. Then came bioinformatics with computer software to classify, manage, and store biological information, and biobanks to store the actual biological specimens—or at least their genes. By this time people were busy coining their own bio- words: biopresents, biofutures, bioproducts, biocracy, biovalue, biolife, biodeath, and others. Each had an idiosyncratic definition, sometimes to develop a new concept, and sometimes just to name a new company—but always to evoke an emotional response. One of the latest bio- words, occurring mostly just in this century, is biohealth.

"Biohealth" encapsulates both the diversity of thinking and the underlying assumptions of the modern Western view of health—a view that is rapidly being diffused worldwide. Who uses "biohealth," where, and how is a fascinating study, for it introduces us to so much of what is new, yet now characteristic, of the way we view health today. Though I could not find the word in any English dictionary, I encountered thousands of entries on internet search engines, and thereby discovered how the word is being used.[3]

The least frequent use I found was as a generic compound word. In education, "biohealth sciences" means "the biological and health sciences." In business, I found a generic reference to "the biohealth/ biotechnology sector"—those companies that make products from the applications of molecular biological research. Likewise "bio-health information resources" was a reference to bioinformatics. I also found the phrase "biohealth of soil," apparently referring to microorganisms in the soil that enhance plant growth. Yet I found none of these specific meanings used very often; apparently there were other adequate ways to say what the new word meant. It is not these generic uses, however, that make the word emblematic of twenty-first-century health; rather, it is the use of the word as a brand name or the title of a company or organization.

---

3. Searching performed in late 2007.

Inje University in Korea hosts the Biohealth Products Research Center, involved in molecular biological research. Hungary's National Committee for Technological Development has a Department of Bio-health and Agricultural Technologies. The Euro-BioHealth Project promotes vocational training for biotechnology and the production of bioproducts. Not surprisingly, commercial companies have also adopted the word in their names, such as the American BioHealth Group LLC, a "targeted disease pharmaceutical company," and Axon Biohealth, a health care and biotechnology company linking the Middle East and North Africa. Worldwide, these projects, centers, departments, and companies all use the same understanding of "biohealth": a word almost synonymous with biotechnology.

Complementary and Alternative Medicine companies and labora-tories have also utilized "biohealth" in their names. Biohealth Labs in Canada makes natural cosmetics, antioxidants, vitamins, and herbal preparations. BioHealth Diagnostics in the US offers "hormone tests" on stool, urine, and saliva mailed in to them, and refers the patient to biohealth practitioners. Astop Biohealth Ltd in Australia makes a prod-uct for asthma prevention containing vitamins and antioxidants. Sky BioHealth Solutions Inc in the US focuses on medications for skin dis-eases, premature aging, and fibromyalgia. And the Bio Health Company in the Netherlands makes the BioHealth Chip for several conditions, worn around the neck with information in its metallic strip said to be activated by skin contact. In response to companies like these, the Biohealth Research Ltd group in Japan was set up to evaluate the claims of commodities like these, and other "nutraceuticals."

Clearly for these latter companies, the word "biohealth" has differ-ent connotations than simply "biotechnology." For them, "bio" is prob-ably meant to suggest "life" or biological medications, and "health" may be drawn from an association with "health foods," or possibly meant to emphasize the broader concept of "health" as opposed to only "medi-cine." These companies seem to have used "biohealth" to suggest very specific associations in the minds of potential clients. Conventional companies and research groups, on the other hand, appear to have taken the stylish "bio-" prefix and attached it onto the more noble word "health" to describe their ongoing work in biotechnology.

A third group of organizations adopting the word bio-health (often with a hyphen) are those involved with bioinformatics. De Montfort

University in the UK hosts the Bio-Health Informatics Research Group, Manchester University in the UK hosts the Bio-Health Informatics Group, and a research partnership in the UK is called the Northwest Institute for BioHealth Informatics (NIBHI). Similarly, Europe Innova has a project called BioHealth, based in Germany, which is involved with eHealth security standards, and NIBHI sponsored a workshop on E-epidemiology called Bio-Health 2006.

Generically, bioinformatics refers to the use of computers to manage any biological data, while eHealth refers specifically to the use of electronic processes in health care (electronic medical records, evidence-based medicine, telemedicine), and E-epidemiology to the use of digital media (internet, mobile phones) in practicing epidemiology. Why, then, would these informatics groups choose the term bio-health? Clearly the application of bioinformatics to health care specifically (rather than, say, to pure research or genetically modified crops) needs a qualifying term. But why not simply health informatics? Perhaps, once again, the reason has more to do with what the word connotes. The "bio-" prefix seems to have become shorthand for advanced medical products and procedures, as in "biomedical" and "biotechnology." And "health" seems to occupy the moral high ground compared with "medicine": we talk of a healthcare (now one word) system rather than a medical care system. Putting the latest medical advances (bio) together with the desired result (health) not only describes the terrain, but also carries emotional weight.

For these same reasons, other organizations have adopted the word. There is a blog for news in the biotech and healthcare industries called BioHealth Investor. There is a consulting firm in the US called BioHealth Management Inc. And in Norway there is a large population-based cohort study of information and specimens (stored in a biobank) called BioHealth Norway.

It is interesting to speculate when biohealth will first appear in a dictionary—and when it does, what definition it will carry! In the meantime, we have a new word, and its current usage indicates a multifaceted picture of what we believe health to be in the twenty-first century:

Biohealth means biotechnology, and that means very specialized and advanced research and pharmaceutical development.

Biohealth also means a rebellion against the dominance of biotechnology. For some people, its use in "holistic" or natural-product companies implies a repudiation of bioscience; for others, simply an entirely different but "complementary" perspective. This means that health does not mean just one thing for all people: approaches to it are (in academic language) "contested knowledges."

Bio-health means computers and all they can do to analyze, manage, store, and transmit information. They are now apparently necessary not only for the development of biotechnology, but for the delivery of healthcare itself.

Biohealth is an industry that can be invested in, a system that needs to be managed, an endeavor that needs security standards, and a reservoir of genetic information stored in a biobank.

Biohealth is international. Its sources are in the industrialized "West"—now including East Asia, Oceana, and the Middle East as well as Europe and North America—and its products, or at least its hopes, are rapidly diffusing into the rest of the world.

And BioHealth (with a capital B and sometimes a capital H) is a brand name, a part of the market economy, a commodity that can—or rather must—be bought. This is accepted by both "conventional" medicine and "alternative" medicine: it is not "contested."

Biohealth, as we shall use the term here, is all of this. However, I would like to suggest a very specific definition for biohealth, for this book at least. The English word "health" means soundness or well-being, coming from a root word meaning whole; the word "holy" comes from the same root. Health is included in the Hebrew concept *shalom*. The World Health Organization definition of health ("a state of complete physical, mental, and social well-being, not merely the absence of disease or infirmity") tries to describe this broader state of wellness. Health, defined this way, has little or no connection with medicine.

Now, though "bio-" merely means life, twentieth-century usage of the bio- prefix has specifically meant the biological sciences, as in "biomedical": applying the findings of the biological sciences to medicine. Using this meaning of bio-, *biohealth means the sort of health or wholeness that results from employing the biological sciences*. All of the aspects of biohealth noted in the above examples fit with this definition.

There is a problem, however. Health means wholeness; qualifying it by "bio-" narrows it to a certain sort of wholeness, that which is brought about by the applications of the biological sciences. Those applications may be very beneficial, but those benefits cannot be called health, because they are not whole. Putting "bio-" in front of "health" limits it—

and limiting wholeness destroys it. Biohealth, a cutting edge futuristic new word, is a contradiction in terms, a reductionism so profound that biohealth comes to mean antihealth.

But we do not mind this, or even notice: we are pleased with the applications of the medical sciences that help us limit or eliminate disease, or even reduce our risk of getting it. This has become a substitute understanding of health for us. We are not bothered by the loss of wholeness because we long ago took wholeness to be only the sum of the parts, most of which we think we understand. We have in fact redefined health to be only biohealth.

In choosing this new word for our contemporary understanding of health in our medical—or medicalized—world, however, it should be clear that I am not uncovering a new concept. Many scholars have, over the last twenty or thirty years, wrestled with what is happening to "health" in our modern world, and several have attached names to it. Twenty-five years ago Arney and Bergen called it "the management of living"[4]; Nikolas Rose more recently called it "the management of life."[5] Robert Kugelmann called it "standardized health" (as opposed to "being-healthy").[6] Clarke et al. coined the term "biomedicalization,"[7] and Ivan Illich called the society where this is in place a "brave new biocracy."[8]

Other scholars have named vital elements of this concept: Robert Crawford referred to "healthism" and a "new health consciousness,"[9] Peterson and Lupton (and others) to "the new public health,"[10] Richard Stivers to "happiness-health as consumption" and "health-happiness as adjustment,"[11] and David Armstrong to "surveillance medicine."[12] All of these contribute to biohealth. However, there is as yet no single commonly agreed on word that scholars from diverse disciplines use for what they are all discussing. I propose "biohealth."

---

4. Arney and Bergen, *Medicine and the Management of Living*.

5. Rose, "Politics of Life," 1.

6. Kugelmann, "Health in Critical Health Psychology," 79–80.

7. Clarke et al., "Biomedicalization," 162.

8. Illich, "Brave New Biocracy."

9. Crawford, Robert, "Health as a Meaningful Social Practice," 407–10.

10. Peterson and Lupton, *New Public Health*.

11. Stivers, *Technology as Magic*, 148.

12. Armstrong, "Rise of Surveillance Medicine," 395.

Biohealth has become a way we think within biomedicine, but it is not the same thing as biomedicine. The focus of biomedicine is on diseased life; the focus of biohealth is on all of life. It is possible, though difficult, to "practice biomedicine" today without "practicing biohealth"; it is possible to think about suffering and healing in other ways, to see them through other lenses than that of biohealth. But the predominant strain of medical thinking today, especially in the industrialized West, has become biohealth thinking. It is woven into everything we do, whether we are patients or practitioners, clients or clinicians. It has become "normal"—but it is not normal.

Our situation is like the frogs playing in a large vat of water gradually heating up over a *very* slow fire. The change in temperature is so gradual, and they "adapt" so well, that they don't realize they are cooking. Put a few frogs into that vat who are not used to it and they immediately leap out, to the surprise of the frogs who are cooking. We who work in biohealth are, unbeknownst to us, cooking.

This book is a systematic look at biohealth. To more fully understand it, we will begin in Part I by looking at its history, and specifically at those developments and trends in biomedicine that allowed for and encouraged the transformation to biohealth. In Part II we will consider several aspects or themes that are the essence of biohealth, the elements that are its foundation and supporting structures. Then in Part III we will look at two case studies of biohealth: Family Medicine, especially in the West, and AIDS treatment in Africa. We will throughout be considering some research and thinking that questions the hegemony of biohealth, and then consider some choices that face us. It is, as I said above, possible to practice, and to be treated with, medicine that does not subscribe to the oxymoron that is biohealth. My hope in this book is to begin the process of return to a sane understanding of health. It is time to jump out of the vat.

PART I

The History of Biohealth

I KNOW THAT HISTORY DOES not proceed with periods like steps in a staircase, each of the same length and significance. History proceeds far more like a path winding through a forest up a mountain, with dips and switchbacks and long, level stretches. Or, using a more dynamic metaphor, like a gusty wind that blows repeatedly under the edges of an old tin roof, gradually loosening the nails, until one day part of the roof blows off. Though it would not be possible to predict when the tin would actually blow off—so much depends on how rusty the nails are, how rotten the wood is, and how much wind there is—it is clear that the day the roof is gone, the house enters a new period of its history. And that new period started abruptly, in the few minutes it took for the roof to lift off.

The history of medicine is much like that path through the woods, though in the last century the path seems more steeply upward, and above the tree-line where the next steps are increasingly visible. It is also a history of wind blowing, where some houses seem to be suddenly de-roofed, and others, though built slowly, are roofed within a day. The sharp turns in the path, the roofings and de-roofings, tempt us to describe that history as a staircase, with definite periods inaugurated by "watershed" events.

In the brief historical overview that follows, I have succumbed to that temptation—partially. I have adopted the three periods that several scholars from varying disciplines have used: the beginning of the twentieth century until World War II, World War II until around 1980, and 1980 to the present.[1] These periods form a convenient outline in

---

1. Illich, *Conviviality*, 1–9 and "Brave New Biocracy," paragraph 55; Relman, "Future

which to locate significant developments and events, to describe trends and processes. And, in retrospect, a few of the developments look suspiciously like watershed events.

The subject matter of the first period (chapter 2) is the development of scientific biomedicine. Clearly the roots of this are in sixteenth-century Renaissance thinking and the developments that followed. Some scholars prefer to date the origin of modern medicine itself at the beginning of the nineteenth century;[2] others at the beginning of the twentieth.[3] The exact starting date is immaterial; what is important is the general agreement that major new developments within modern biomedicine occurred in the first half of the twentieth century. What is equally important is that many of these scholars date the end of this period (and the beginning of the next) at around World War II.[4]

This general agreement that something fundamentally changed in modern medicine after World War II (chapter 3) carries several descriptions. Some are clearly laudatory, speaking, for example, of the "phenomenal" "post-war therapeutic revolution" leading to "The Rise" in modern medicine.[5] Some scholars describe similar phenomena—"the explosive development of new medical technology," together with "specialism" and "the rise of medical insurance"[6]—but with less obvious, or at least mixed, praise. And to some, the "new medical revolution"[7] brought with it increased control of our lives, increased "medicalization,"[8] and even "sickening side effects"[9] and "counterproductivity."[10] This post-war

of Medical Practice" and Clarke, "Biomedicalization," 163–64, have all proposed variants of these three periods. Elsewhere, Clarke, "From the Rise," 2, provides a table succinctly summarizing her view of these three periods.

2. Arney and Bergen, *Medicine and the Management of Living,* 46; Crawford, "Health as a Meaningful Social Practice," 405.

3. Clarke, "Biomedicalization," 163; Fox, *Power and Illness,* 30ff.; Relman, "Future of Medical Practice," 6; Illich, *Conviviality,* 1,

4. Clarke, "Biomedicalization," 163; Fox, *Power and Illness,* 56ff; Arney and Bergen, *Medicine and the Management of Living,* 46; Illich, *Conviviality,* 2, 6; Relman, "Future of Medical Practice," 8.

5. Le Fanu, *Rise and Fall of Modern Medicine,* 160.

6. Relman, "Future of Medical Practice," 8–10.

7. Arney and Bergen, *Medicine and the Management of Living,* 46.

8. Clarke, "Biomedicalization," 163–64.

9. Illich, *Conviviality,* 2.

10. Illich, *Medical Nemesis,* 211ff.

period coincides with changes in our world economy and even more fundamental changes in our relationship with nature and each other. Jacques Ellul described three historical periods for humanity: the prehistoric period (until 3,000 BC), the historic period (until WWII), and the post-historic period (beginning with WWII). He also called this latter period The Technological Society.[11]

What is equally astonishing is to see the general agreement among scholars that something else happened to (or within) medicine around 1980, the beginning of our third period. What developed in this period is the essence of what I have called biohealth, and in chapter 4 we will consider changes within our societies that introduced this period, followed by the characteristics of biohealth itself in Part II. Here, I want only to demonstrate from several perspectives the focus on the years around 1980. Le Fanu, the one who saw the "Rise" in modern medicine, saw "The Fall" beginning "from the early 1980s onwards."[12] Writing in the early 1980s, Relman saw commercialism and a new medical-industrial complex overwhelming American medicine, at least.[13] Fox saw American health policy moving from "compromise" to "disarray" in 1975.[14] Arney said that "by 1980," medicine was affirming "systems theory" in its self-understanding.[15] Clarke et al., who describe the previous period as "medicalization," say that "beginning about 1985 . . . the nature of medicalization itself began to change," resulting in what they call "biomedicalization"[16]—having characteristics that overlap with what I am calling biohealth.

However, there is a problem with dividing history into neat periods, each with its own title and watershed events. When we impose an outline onto history, it begins to make the path through the forest look like a staircase. We may even begin to think that the watershed events caused the subsequent history, rather than simply heralding it. The point, then, is not that these periods are "real"; history remains far messier. Medicalization, for example, existed in the first period and continued into the third; biomedical developments clearly did not stop at the end

---

11. Stivers, *Technology as Magic*, 17, 22ff.

12. Le Fanu, *Rise and Fall of Modern Medicine*, 235.

13. Relman, "Future of Medical Practice," 13–16.

14. Fox, *Power and Illness*, 84ff.

15. Arney and Bergen, *Medicine and the Management of Living*, 47, 72ff.

16. Clarke, "Biomedicalization," 164ff.

of the first period. The events and trends, however, really did happen, meaning that the medical world we live in today, formed by these events, is very different from the medical world of our great-grandparents—or even our parents. Considering the effect of those events and trends on our medical world should help us understand biohealth better. And when we understand it, we can more wisely live with it.

2

Biomedicine: 1900 to World War II

A USEFUL HISTORY OF BIOMEDICINE would begin long before 1900, likely some time in the sixteenth century. Over the following three centuries there was sufficient theoretical foundation laid, so that by the nineteenth century we can see the development of pivotal technologies that we still use: the stethoscope, the ophthalmoscope, the spirometer for pulmonary function tests, general anesthesia, surgical antisepsis, and the bacteriological work of Koch and Pasteur. By the end of the century we knew the cause of malaria (1898), we had x-rays (1895) and the electrocardiograph (1901).[1] Before our first time period begins, biomedicine was already recognizable as biomedicine.

The year 1900 must have been an interesting time to be a doctor: we had the capability of extensive clinical diagnosis, using the diagnostic tools just mentioned, and the ability to confirm diagnoses, and even correct some problems, with surgery. But there were few truly effective medicines then. In 1900, William Osler, the great clinician, was a professor at Johns Hopkins University; he said, "One of the first duties of the physician is to educate the masses not to take medicine." And this: "The young physician starts life with 20 drugs for each disease, and the old physician ends life with one drug for 20 diseases."[2] While there is still wisdom in these sentiments, their importance today is in reflecting the medical world he knew. Other than morphine, a few hypnotics, digitalis, nitroglycerine, quinine, aspirin, smallpox vaccine, emetine for amebic

1. Reiser, *Medicine and Technology*.

2. BrainyQuote, William Osler. Online: http://www.brainyquote.com/quotes/authors/w/william_osler.html.

dysentery, and the recently introduced thyroid extract, along with lemons to treat scurvy and cod liver oil to treat rickets,[3] he was bereft of a safe "therapeutic armamentarium."

A dozen drugs. Yet by the end of this first historical period, the American FDA (itself another development of this period) had approved over 4,000 drugs, and by 1980 nearly ten thousand.[4] This observation alone may be justification enough to define a time period beginning in 1900. Biomedicine was ready then to begin being effective. Effectiveness, if fact, is precisely the characteristic Ivan Illich used in his description of this first historical period (which he defined as 1913–1955). He proposed that any industrial institution begins with a period of applying science to solve problems, and does so successfully. He claimed, however, that every such institution—transportation, education, social work, medicine—then enters a period of counter-productivity, where the successes begin to be counter-balanced by side effects of the technology itself.[5] Nevertheless, in the first half of the century, biomedicine began building, and building rapidly, on the nineteenth-century discoveries noted above. Biomedicine grew and continues to grow because biomedicine works.

Surgery certainly works, but its main barriers, pain and infection, had already been addressed in the nineteenth century. It was in the first half of the twentieth century, then, when pharmacology blossomed. Insulin was isolated in 1921, diphtheria, pertussis, tetanus, and BCG vaccines were all developed in the 1920s, sulfa antibiotics began being used in the 1930s, and penicillin, though first discovered in 1928, was finally used successfully in 1942. Within a brief twenty-year span, we had doubled the number of vaccines available, developed safe cures for infections, and transformed diabetes from a fatal disease to a chronic one. Or, to say it more generally, we could now dependably prevent some diseases by giving medication, cure some others by giving medication, and we could keep some people alive and mostly healthy by having them take medication for the rest of their lives.

These pharmaceutical advances complemented ongoing work in medical technology and surgery. The iron lung was developed in 1927, a precursor of contemporary "life support" technology, and research had

---

3. Bálint et al., "Sir William Osler," 51–53.

4. FDA website.

5. Illich, *Conviviality*, 1–9.

already begun on artificial kidneys and the heart-lung bypass machine. And surgery continued to advance, aided by discoveries in physiology and the development of blood banks in 1935. The idea of replacing (and later transplanting) organs became a reality in 1938 with the development of the artificial hip. By the end of the first half of the century, biomedicine was not just a hope or promise of effectiveness, it was actually effective, and was promising even further effectiveness.

These technological developments are hallmarks of this period we've called *biomedicine*. Yet they are not the only events we need to be aware of as we consider its eventual transformation to *biohealth*. Biotechnological advances are the foundation on which biohealth is built, but there were also social and political developments during this period that were vital for the eventual appearance of biohealth. We will now consider in more detail six developments in this period that paved the way for biohealth.

FLEXNER REPORT 1910

The Flexner Report published in 1910 is often regarded as a turning point in American medicine, a reform document that tightened up American medical education and assured the firm scientific foundation on which biomedicine, and now biohealth, are built. It certainly provides us with an event and a year that symbolize an important change in American medicine—but as Paul Starr points out,[6] the change in medicine was far more gradual, with many factors beyond the Flexner report.

In the nineteenth century, before biomedicine had proven itself, there were many competing views of how to heal, none able to conclusively prove its worth compared with the others. As we have seen, the roots of the biomedical approach had already been established, but the fruits had not yet developed. Homeopathy was one competing approach, but there were others that have since disappeared. Each approach had its own schools. But in addition to competing approaches, there was also a profusion of proprietary medical schools, essentially diploma mills, that were completely unregulated and produced poor quality doctors. Altogether, there were 162 medical schools in the US in 1906.

6. Starr, *Social Transformation*, 93–127.

Several reforms at the beginning of the twentieth century attacked these problems, reforms that included state licensing boards as well as the Flexner Report, which proposed standards for medical education. All together they had a dramatic effect. By the time Flexner's Report was published, thirty-one medical schools had already closed for failing to meet licensing requirements. By 1915, another thirty-six had closed, and by 1922 the number open was down to eighty-one, exactly half of the number sixteen years earlier. During these years homeopathic schools either closed or became allopathic schools.

The reform efforts, licensing, and the Flexner Report were clearly successful in setting standards, resulting in massive medical school closures. And it appears that the targets were twofold: the unscrupulous diploma mills and the medical "sectarians." Clamping down on dishonest, inadequate schools, while necessary, did not change the direction of biomedicine; but choosing one approach over all the competing approaches did change the direction—or at least eliminate competition from alternative directions. In between these two poles was the simple matter of mandating a longer training period and adequate laboratories, both of which solidified the scientific biomedical approach, which is the foundation of biohealth.

Sectarian approaches didn't disappear—in fact, chiropractic and osteopathy were just beginning—but they developed outside of the mainstream (though osteopathy has subsequently "joined"). By 1930, all non-biomedical practitioners together took care of only 5 percent of patients. But this "victory" of biomedicine over alternative approaches to healing was only apparent, and ultimately short-lived. Of course not all patients benefit from, or even appreciate, the offerings of biomedicine; it cannot always deliver. But that only exposes the brilliance of biohealth: built firmly on a biomedical foundation, it nonetheless embraces alternatives—or rather they embrace it, as we saw in the introductory chapter.

INTERNATIONAL CLASSIFICATION OF DISEASES (ICD) 1900

Flexner and the accompanying state licensing boards said, among other things, that scientifically based medicine was to be the only legitimate medicine. They officially sanctioned, and therefore enthroned, biomedicine. This science of biomedicine followed the analytic approach of Descartes, which was to analyze smaller and smaller parts of something as a means of understanding the whole. That was, and still is, a very successful method for discovering the mechanisms of disease, and then discovering the mechanisms of repair. There was in addition, however, another method of scientific study less dramatic than dissection and microscopy, but poised to equal them in importance and eventually carry them on its back: statistics. In 1900, a decade before Flexner, the International Classification of Diseases (ICD) was launched. It was not the birth of biostatistics, but it was a hallmark event signaling its importance.

Classifying disease was not new in 1900, nor was the use of statistics in studying disease. Seventy years earlier Pierre Charles Alexandre Louis in Paris had used statistical analysis in looking systematically at tuberculosis and typhoid, and later by the same method had shown the inefficacy of bloodletting as a treatment. And almost fifty years before ICD, John Snow had used epidemiological analysis to demonstrate that a cholera outbreak in London could be traced to the Broad Street water pump, and he stopped the epidemic by removing the handle of the pump. By 1900, however, it had become clear that in order to use statistics internationally, it would be necessary to standardize diagnosing internationally. It was also becoming clear that statistical analysis was necessary to broaden our understanding of disease in this larger international "data-base." To build our Tower of Biomedicine, we needed to all speak the same language. The ICD gave us that language.

Disease classification and its analysis is certainly a very powerful tool for understanding disease in populations—and is consequently one of the foundations of biohealth. Yet, like so many of the developments in this chapter, its very power can blind us to its deficiencies. Consider classification in general: classifications are very useful for physical characteristics that can be measured. Stones can be classified according to color or weight, tree leaves according to shape, people according to gender or height or eye color. Some disease entities in people can also be easily classified: a baby can be born alive or dead, an injury can have a bone fracture or not, a person's difficulty in breathing can be accompanied by a fever or not. The same disease, though, does not always present the same way in all people, and the pain that accompanies many diseases is notoriously difficult to measure. Those periodically revising ICD have responded to these difficulties by increasing the number of codes—from less than two hundred in 1900 to tens of thousands today. Increasing the number of codes theoretically makes room for everything—assuming the data is accurately recorded.

It is, however, not always accurately recorded. Errors in recording average around 20 percent, but in some studies are as high as 50 percent or more.[7] That is a high error rate for a tool that has had a century to perfect itself. But even if the problem of errors was solved, there is a more fundamental problem: assuming that all dis-ease can be codified and compared internationally. What do we do with chronic fatigue syndrome in Africa, or neurasthenia in the United States? Even within the homeland of biomedicine—Europe and North America—we still have major differences in the way we diagnose and treat disease.[8] Yet even if we eliminated all errors in recording and agreed worldwide on disease classification, we still must deal with the conundrum of coding itself.

This problem of transforming a human dis-ease into a numerical code shows up especially when data is computerized. Because computer software provides us with standardized categories, it is "all but impossible to enter certain kinds of data," and "all but impossible *not* to record other kinds of data."[9] In other words, the coding system presents us with a certain way to think about disease, even if that way differs from our experience. Instead of the lived reality of the disease setting the agenda of the way we think, the coding system does.

Now these critiques are merely descriptive; none completely invalidates the successful use of statistics in understanding disease in populations. In fact, this very success gradually induced biomedicine to use statistics in the diagnosis and treatment of individual people. "There's a 60 percent chance these drugs will cure your cancer." "The Doc says Grampa has three months to live." We have come to depend on numbers, to feel more satisfied with "a 60 percent chance" than "it's a toss-up." This numerical approach characterizes biohealth. We could have no risk analysis, no evidence-based medicine without the approach ushered in by the ICD. Biohealth depends so heavily on these tools, as we shall see, that questions of disease-meaning, of *healing* even, are sometimes squeezed off of its agenda. And again we see the brilliance

7. O'Malley et al., "Measuring Diagnoses," 1620–39.

8. Payer, *Medicine and Culture.*

9. Clarke et al., "Biomedicalization," 174.

of biohealth: it does to healing what it does with Complementary and Alternative Medicine. It makes room for them within itself, gives them names ("CAM," "spirituality," "pastoral care"), studies their effectiveness—statistically of course—and then compares that effectiveness with itself. It co-opts them, and then "proves" they are not as effective as it is.

MARGARET SANGER AND MARIE STOPES 1916

Margaret Sanger in the US and Marie Stopes in the UK are generally known for their contributions to the development of birth control and their advocacy for women's rights to control their own bodies. Margaret Sanger founded Planned Parenthood, and the work of Marie Stopes is carried on in a parallel organization, Marie Stopes International. They are also both known for their support for a social movement, popular at the time, called eugenics. Their leadership in family planning is lauded even today by those who are concerned about world population growth and women's rights. Likewise their support of eugenics is castigated today by those who see in eugenics an incipient Nazism requiring the destruction of innocent human life.

Margaret Sanger came to prominence in 1916 when she opened the first birth-control clinic in New York City—and was subsequently arrested and spent thirty days in jail. At that time in the US disseminating contraceptive information and devices was considered obscene and was illegal. Two years later Marie Stopes in the UK published her first book, *Married Love*, and later opened a birth-control clinic in London. Both women were troubled on seeing poor urban families with many children, and felt their poverty would be eased if they had fewer children. This fit well with their insistence that all women should be able to control their own bodies, including childbearing.

In addition to this social concern (neither woman, by the way, was poor), both also felt that "negative" human characteristics, both physical and attitudinal, were inherited. It was this belief that was behind the program of the eugenics movement: that those who were "unfit" (a broad category including certainly the mentally retarded, but often also criminals, the immoral, the poor, immigrants, and Blacks) should be sterilized, often involuntarily. In the 1920s and 30s, nearly half of US states had forced sterilization laws, and many thousands, especially in institutions, were sterilized. There was a parallel emphasis, though less prominent with Sanger and Stopes, that those who were "fit" (i.e., those from the upper and middle classes) needed to procreate more. In fact, part of eugenic thinking was a sense of "genetic responsibility," that people had a duty to their society, or more specifically to their nation or race, to make reproductive choices that would promote a healthy population, and consequently resist genetic degeneration.[10] This underlying concern of eugenics, to improve or even "cleanse" the national gene pool, was behind the Nazi holocaust.

The connection of eugenics with Nazism is enough to discredit the movement for most people. In addition, for those opposed to abortion, the notion of aborting fetuses with congenital anomalies again raises the specter of eugenics. And for people suspicious of why those in the developed world want those in the developing (brown and black) world to have fewer children, the eugenics specter is again raised. But look more closely: our problems with eugenics are not with its fundamental premise—that disease can be transmitted genetically, and that we should intervene genetically. Rather, our problems are in deciding that whole groups could be considered "unfit," and in involuntarily sterilizing or aborting or killing those we have declared unfit. In the 1920s, people wanted to improve the genes of a human population by selective breeding. Today people want to improve the genes of an individual by genetic engineering. Our methods today are sometimes more voluntary, but our goal has not changed.

"Eugenics" simply means "good birth"—clearly a goal of medicine in any generation. Both eugenics and genetic engineering want to give every person a good birth by controlling their genetic makeup. Though they have different approaches, their goal is the same. We need to evaluate eugenics not only by the methods it chooses, but also by this goal. Or turn it upside-down: we need to evaluate genetic engineering not simply by its lack of *imposed* genetic manipulations, but by its eugenic goal of changing and controlling the genetic make-up of a person, or of that person's offspring.

This is important for biohealth. Biohealth would repudiate any link with forced or compulsory *anything*. People in biohealth are free, autonomous. And because of this, biohealth encourages responsibility for one's own health, as we shall see—in the same way that eugenics encour-

10. Crawford, "Health as a Meaningful Social Practice," 406.

aged genetic responsibility. And biohealth, embracing the biosciences to facilitate health, embraces the *control* of the body that biomedicine requires. Margaret Sanger promoted a pivotal example: birth *control*. The irony, not immediately apparent, is this: while biohealth insists that we have responsibility for our own health, we end up relinquishing the control of our health to the system of biohealth. We will explore this further in Part II.

INSULIN 1921

I am strongly tempted to make the following audacious statement: chronic disease was born on January 23, 1922, the day Leonard Thompson received his first successful injection of insulin, and went on to live thirteen more years as an insulin-dependent diabetic. What tempts me is the almost fairy-tale story of the discovery of insulin and its profound effect on biohealth.

The story[11] takes place in Toronto, Canada—further evidence, if needed, that biohealth is truly international. Frederick Banting, thirty years old and just a year out of his surgical internship, had a rough start financially in his private practice, and took up a part time job at a medical school. While there, he had a few ideas for some experiments on dogs to isolate the pancreatic factor that controlled blood sugar. Dr. J. R. R. Macleod at the University of Toronto reluctantly gave him laboratory space in the Department of Physiology, together with an assistant, twenty-two-year-old Charles Best, who had just taken his undergraduate degree in physiology and biochemistry. After a few months work in early 1921, they had isolated insulin and began giving it to dogs with surgically removed pancreases. By the end of the year they gave it orally to a new diabetic person, but it had no effect. J. B. Collip, twenty-nine years old and with a recent graduate degree in biochemistry, joined them to work on an injectable extract, and it was his extract that worked on Leonard Thompson and kept him alive for thirteen more years.

One year later over a thousand diabetic patients were using insulin. One of them, treated by Banting himself, was five years old, and eventually lived seventy years on insulin. By the end of that year, 1923, Banting and Macleod were awarded the Nobel Prize in Medicine for their

11. University of Toronto Library website.

work—and Banting (the first Canadian to receive the prize—Macleod was Scottish), recognizing the contributions of Best, shared half of his prize with him. Likewise Macleod shared half his prize with Collip.

Even the follow-up stories continue the fairy tale. Banting was the immediate celebrity, but the only one whose significant scientific contribution ended with insulin. His first marriage ended after eight years, but he remained humble despite being knighted in 1934, and he remained patriotic. He had served in World War I and was wounded then; he joined the military again in World War II and was killed in an accidental plane crash in 1941. Macleod had been an authority on carbohydrate metabolism prior to the discovery of insulin; he continued researching and writing. Best took further degrees and eventually went on to become Chair of Physiology at the University of Toronto, the post previously occupied by Macleod, who recommended him. He and Collip, the two not officially recognized in the Nobel Prize, ended up with the most successful lives in academia and research.

The insulin story makes a wonderful poster child for biomedicine. The principals are young, not American, and seem remarkably free of ego-driven arrogance. Even their flaws add to the charm: Collip neglected to write down the formula for his first successful insulin extract and it took him three months to rediscover it; Banting's failed marriage may have been in part due to the sudden celebrity of a humble patriotic farm boy. This is the system of biomedical discovery at its best: from an idea scribbled in a notebook while preparing a lecture to a Nobel Prize in just three years. And unlike some biomedical discoveries, such as the new antidepressants or Botox or cosmetic surgery, there is no controversy about insulin, no questionable uses, no drug company half-truths.

Now look again. My audacious statement was that *chronic disease* was born on January 23, 1922. Let us first dispense with the silliness in that statement. Chronic disease has obviously been with us as long as any disease has, for any disability (blindness, arthritis) is a chronic disease: it is chronic because it does not go away. But there is another sort of chronic disease that insulin ushered in, the sort that becomes chronic precisely because there is a drug that keeps the person from dying. Before insulin, Type I diabetes was acute, and then fatal; insulin transformed it into a chronic disease. Most recently we have done the same with AIDS using ARVs. This sort of chronic disease depends on something in the medical system, usually drugs, to keep it from becoming a fatal disease—and therefore the patient must be a permanent patient, with a lifelong dependency on the medical system.

We should not underestimate what a major change this has been in the history of medicine, nor should we overlook how recently this has occurred. Other than thyroid extract developed only two decades earlier, medical care did not have the concept of taking medicines for one's whole life *in order to stay alive.* In his day, Osler was quite right to encourage people *not* to take medicines. Humanity does not have a cultural memory of this lifelong need to take daily medicines to avoid death; it has occurred only within the lifetime of some of our elders who are still alive today. Blind people, deaf people, lame people—none of these historically depended on the medical system; they depended on their communities. It is one thing for the medical community to understand and promote dependence on itself; it is a far larger task to imbue this in the human consciousness. The world-wide difficulty of chronic disease patients adhering to their treatment programs is ample evidence of this.

Diabetes was the first disease to test this approach on a large scale; insulin was the first development that made this possible. Now, as with the scientific basis of medicine or the use of statistics, or even eugenics in its pure form, the task here is only to see the historical setting of insulin and the rest of these developments, not censure them. None of these developments are purely "good" or "bad." Insulin is certainly lifesaving, and clearly has given many people who would otherwise be dead a relatively normal life. At the same time, insulin was a harbinger of an entirely new category of disease that it "created."

Yet insulin was only one of the forces that "created" chronic disease. The actual pattern of diseases in the developed world was changing as well, partly because infectious diseases were declining and being replaced by the so-called diseases of affluence. In 1927 the *Index Medicus* first included an entry for "Diseases, chronic"; by 1947 we find "Chronic illness"; and not until 1957 the current heading of "Chronic disease."[12] However, another possible reason for the "epidemic" of chronic diseases was simply the way we study disease—and, again, our use of statistics: "It was the creation of the sociomedical survey that brought chronic illness to the attention of researchers; . . . it was the perpetual collection of statistical data that led to its birth as a concept."[13] Whatever the reason,

12. Armstrong, "Genealogical Method," 1225–27.
13. Galvin, "Disturbing Notions of Chronic Illness," 114.

today chronic disease care is at the heart of biohealth. Biohealth claims for those with chronic diseases the same as it claims for all pre-patients: a "healthy" life for those who follow its dictates.

DPT VACCINE 1923–1927

In a way, vaccines do not belong here at all. Their origin, with Edward Jenner using cowpox to vaccinate against smallpox, was a hundred and thirty years earlier than DPT. Then during the late nineteenth century, based on the findings of Pasteur and Koch, there were four more vaccines developed—for rabies, typhoid, cholera, and plague. Immunization by vaccines— the idea of inoculating a person with a small amount of something to prevent them from getting a disease—was not a product of the twentieth century. In fact, the science underlying the development of further vaccines was expanding rapidly as the century opened. The first Nobel Prize in Medicine was awarded to Emil von Behring in 1901 for his work in developing an antitoxin to treat diphtheria, and his work laid the foundation for the later development of the diphtheria vaccine.

However, the use of all of these vaccines was not very widespread by 1900. Vaccines were used for those especially at risk of these diseases, soldiers in combat; for example, or to attempt to prevent an outbreak in a community if the disease was nearby. But the need for *all people* to take vaccines regardless of their risk had not yet entered the human consciousness. The contribution of the vaccine developments of the 1920s made possible the widespread acceptance of that *need*, yet another cornerstone of biohealth.

The story of the development of the diphtheria, pertussis, and tetanus vaccines—ultimately the DPT we still use—provides a marked contrast to the discovery of insulin. The insulin story was more like the Jenner story: few memorable famous characters, a clear story line, a single obvious benefit. The DPT story has a larger cast, each having a bit part, with big egos colliding; it begins to suggest a picture of an enterprise so large that no one person could do all the research—or even understand it all—and make all the discoveries. This story of one discovery building rapidly on another, each by a different team, is paradigmatic of modern biomedical research.

The players in this case were German, French, Danish, Japanese, Russian, and English, and the result was a diphtheria vaccine in 1923, pertussis in 1926, and tetanus in 1927—with an American team finally combining the three in 1942. The result was a single injection, to be given three times in infancy and again before starting school, recommended for *all human beings*. An astonishing recommendation, really, putting a pharmaceutical product in the same category as food, water, and air. Yet this is no conspiracy, no plot by a hidden centralized world power to control humanity. This is the evidence of objective science speaking; not a government or an emperor, but a way of thinking that wears "proof" openly as its identifying uniform.

And at first glance the proof seems compelling. At the beginning of the twentieth century, every year over one hundred thousand people in the US alone contracted diphtheria, an equal number pertussis, and over a thousand yearly got tetanus. By the end of the century, diphtheria was virtually unknown, tetanus rare, and pertussis confined to outbreaks a fraction of the size of outbreaks a century earlier.[14] In fact, graphs of diseases such as diphtheria show a sharp decline after immunization is introduced. But interestingly, there was a more substantial decline *before* the introduction of vaccine.[15] The same is true for many infectious diseases: there was a major fall in death rates from nineteenth-century sanitary reforms, before either antibiotics or vaccinations.[16]

And now, finally, we come to a factor that does *not* characterize biohealth. Biohealth embraces procedures and pharmaceuticals of any sort, whether preventive (such as vaccines) or curative, conventional, or "alternative." Biohealth even embraces alternative healing systems— but it is mostly silent about approaches such as the nineteenth-century sanitary reforms. It remains profoundly suspicious of politics, of large-scale social movements that do not promote its products. If biohealth is the sort of wholeness that results from employing the technology of the biological sciences, an approach to health without this technology falls outside of biohealth. Biohealth advocates for and promotes individual acceptance of its products, or even individual behavior change, but it does not embrace the dictum "health becomes a social science."[17] Not

14. CDC website, 2008.

15. McKeown, *Role of Medicine*, 99.

16. Dubos, *Mirage of Health*, 150–51.

17. Wilkinson, *Unhealthy Societies*, chap. 2.

surprisingly, social scientists provide some of the sharpest critiques of biomedicine, and by implication biohealth (see chapter 3).

Look a bit more closely at this suspicion of politics and social control. Biohealth thinking puts the responsibility for good health squarely on the shoulders of each individual, as we shall see in Part II, and consequently is a natural fit for American culture. But many health systems, most in fact, are not as radically individualistic as America's. Do the centrally controlled national health systems of Europe, for example, also subscribe to biohealth thinking? They do, showing once again the malleability and brilliance of biohealth. National health systems are far more efficient than free enterprise ones—efficient, that is, in making the offerings of biohealth available to the entire population, and not just the rich, and in eliminating waste. This is no small matter, for the benefits of biohealth can be measured, and European systems often have better results statistically than the American system, at a far cheaper price. Biohealth remains silent in the face of centrally controlled movements aimed at achieving health without its products, but welcomes national health systems whose main offering is biohealth itself.

Now look just a bit deeper still. Biohealth promotes individual choice, and with it individual responsibility; it eschews obvious coercion. But its power, and the resulting coercion, is far more subtle. There are no laws in biohealth, no health police; there is no need for them. People generally *believe* that vaccines are more dependable in preventing disease than hygiene, that anti-cholesterol drugs are more important than diet, that babies must be born in hospitals in order to survive, that the return from sickness to health of necessity will involve medicines, whether conventional or "complementary and alternative." Coercion is not necessary when people coerce themselves based on beliefs that are at best only partially true. Biohealth first deceives us, and based on this deception we "choose" its offerings: a very clever form of control.[18]

PAP SMEAR 1941

Finally we come to screening for asymptomatic disease, epitomized by the Pap Smear developed by George Papanicolaou before World War II. At first, the Pap Smear story seems more like the simple discovery

18. See Downing, *Death and Life in America*, chap. 3.

of insulin than the complex DPT development we just considered. Dr. George Papanicolaou, a Greek MD-PhD educated in Greece and Germany, began working at New York's Cornell Medical School in 1914 in the Department of Anatomy. In the 1920s he began studying abnormal vaginal cytology as a way of detecting early cancer (published in 1928), and in 1939 began working with a gynecologic pathologist to refine his studies.[19] In 1941 they published their findings in the *American Journal of Obstetrics and Gynecology*.[20] The Pap Smear was born—and with it, the concept of discovering dangerous disease in people who felt fine and considered themselves disease-free.

There are, however, two footnotes to this apparently simple story. The first is that, technically, George Papanicolaou was not the first to describe abnormal cervical cytology as a precursor for cervical cancer. A Romanian pathologist, Aureli Babes, published his 1926 work[21] the year before Papanicolaou first published his.[22] Yet other than the name (I suppose we should be relieved that we don't have a test for young women called the Babes Test), the interesting point is that neither the findings of Babes nor Papanicolaou were noticed and acted on by the medical world in the 1920s. The technology was known and published by two independent investigators, but lay dormant for fifteen years until Papanicolaou again published. Perhaps both scientists were "ahead of their time"; perhaps there were, and still are today, factors other than "pure evidence" that are needed to convince scientists and eventually the public to adopt new technologies. But then again, perhaps it is not so mysterious. Insulin had immediate effects on very ill patients. Screening tests and vaccines need large and long-term studies to prove their dramatic effectiveness.

The other footnote brings us back to an earlier discussion. Papanicolaou published his first paper on cytological screening in the Proceedings of the Third Race Betterment Conference, held in Battle Creek, Michigan, in 1928. As the name implies, the Race Betterment Foundation, which sponsored three conferences in 1914, 1915, and 1928, subscribed to eugenic principles, and was led by John Kellogg,

19. Papanicolaou. Online: http://www.essortment.com/uterinecancerp_ruxf.html
20. Papanicolaou and Traut, "The Diagnostic Value of Vaginal Smears."
21. Babes, "Diagnostic du cancer," 451.
22. Papanicolaou, "New Cancer Diagnosis," 528.

a doctor and inventor of the corn flake.[23] So what possible connection could there be between cytological screening and eugenics?

To propose a connection, it is once again important to look carefully at eugenics. As a movement, it is discredited today for obvious reasons: its main advocates were Anglo-Saxons, and the race they wanted to "better" was the white race, a movement that reached its apogee in Nazism. In addition, their methods included forced sterilizations and ultimately genocide. Choosing one race, and using involuntary methods, are unacceptable to most everyone today—and were unacceptable to some even when the movement was popular.[24]

However, we previously suggested another characteristic of eugenics, that of *control*, that has not fallen out of favor. How would we feel if eugenics reinvented itself today, changed its name, chose the entire human race as the race it wanted to better, and eliminated all involuntary methods? We are not left with nothing; we are left with a goal of getting to the core of our medical problems and giving everyone the possibility of a good birth. This is biohealth. We are no longer controlling people and their bodies without their consent; we are controlling them with full "informed consent." We would not be waiting until people come with advanced disease for which we can do nothing; we would encourage them to come before they even feel ill, because then we have a better chance of controlling the disease process.

And now we begin to get a glimpse of why a eugenics foundation might be interested in cytological screening. At the core of eugenics is not merely the unethical and even evil methods it used. Its core was to utilize the burgeoning scientific discoveries of the early twentieth century for the betterment of people: precisely the goal of biohealth. It realized that control of disease was related to control of people, and that control was easier and more successful if the disease was found in an early, treatable (or controllable) form—and if people embraced that control.

This is neither a polemic for nor against a refashioned eugenics. It is simply an attempt to see in eugenics some of the roots of contemporary biohealth. We may ultimately have reason to critique screening specifically, or biohealth generally, but not because they are eugenics disguised and may lead some day to a Nazi-like control of our lives. I am

---

23. Durst, "Evangelical Engagements with Eugenics."
24. Chesterton, *Eugenics and Other Evils.*

not concerned about what *might happen* in biomedical health care; I am concerned about what is already here in biohealth.

SUMMARY

Of all of the dramatic advances of biomedicine in the first half of the twentieth century, this may initially seem a strange list to represent this period. Many would accept the Flexner report, the discovery of insulin, and perhaps the DPT vaccines as "definitive moments"[25] of this period. But isn't the discovery of penicillin far more important than the activism of Sanger and Stopes? Don't the developments in surgery such as the first artificial hip in 1938 outweigh the Pap smear? Is the creation of the ICD really more important than, say, the development of the US Food and Drug Administration? Why this particular list?

Certainly, if our task were to review the definitive moments of biomedicine, we would need to include antibiotics and surgical advances—and include developments from the nineteenth century. However, the purpose of this chapter, as previously mentioned, is not simply biomedical history, but rather a look at those biomedical developments that are unique to our age and pave the way for biohealth. Look briefly at antibiotic therapy: while certainly dramatically effective in curing infections, antibiotics do not introduce a new style or form of treatment, only a new substance. Herbalists have always functioned the same way, giving substances to patients for a limited amount of time. Treating chronic diseases with lifelong medicines, however, is an entirely new paradigm, unknown in history. Looking, then, at the biomedical developments chronicled here, we can deduce from them several themes.

Science

Flexner and the movement he symbolizes were prescient on at least two accounts: standard-setting, and a scientific foundation. Medicine at the turn of the century was a hodge-podge not only of philosophies of healing, but also of standards. Unethical for-profit diploma mills needed regulation, and bioscience provided a very effective foundation for this

---

25. Le Fanu, *Rise and Fall of Modern Medicine,* chose ten parallel definitive moments for the post-war period.

regulation, as well as for progress. It bears repeating: biomedical science maintains hegemony because it works.

It also is true, and will be repeated, that biomedical science need not be the *only* approach to healing. Social scientists critique biomedicine because it can ignore social causes of ill health, as we will see in the next chapter. There are also cultural factors to health and disease, political factors,[26] and spiritual factors.[27] Biohealth tries to make room for all of these; nevertheless, the foundation, the touchstone, and the definitive judge—and ultimately the limiting factor—of everything that biohealth does is science.

Chronic Disease

We suggested at the end of the insulin story that one possible reason for the growth of chronic diseases in the first half of the twentieth century was the availability of treatments like insulin that changed fatal diseases into chronic diseases. Or this "growth" could have been partly artifactual, due to our increased use of surveys and statistics. Nevertheless, the high prevalence of chronic disease, especially in industrialized countries, is today indisputable. In light of this, one author begins an analysis of the "failure " of American health policy with these words: "The contemporary disarray in health affairs in the United States . . . is the cumulative result of inattention to the burden of chronic disabling illness." "For three-quarters of a century," he says later, "the people who made health policy in the United States accorded priority to acute episodes of illness, [accommodating] the disabling consequences of illness and injury within this priority."[28] The same, I think, applies to any society whose foundational medical system is biomedical. Biomedicine's greatest victories were with acute illnesses and accidents. One reason we may have ignored chronic diseases earlier in the twentieth century is simply that we had less to offer them.

However, biomedicine no longer ignores chronic disease. In fact, "primary care" in the West is almost synonymous with chronic disease care. Much contemporary biomedical research concerns drugs and procedures for organs and body parts that are wearing out. We of course

---

26. Fanon, "Medicine and Colonialism."

27. Downing, *Death and Life in America.*

28. Fox, *Power and Illness*, 1, 113.

"cure" very few of these chronic conditions, so our attention is on life-long medical management. And the first chance we had to do this on a large scale was treating diabetics with insulin.

Population Health

"Population health" and "population medicine" are terms that did not appear in the medical literature until the 1960s. Even now the term "population medicine" is used more in veterinary articles than in medical ones; the two Departments of Population Medicine in North America are both in Veterinary Schools (Cornell, New York, and Guelph, Ontario). And the first few review articles on population health listed in PubMed appeared in the 1980s—in Russian. Clearly biomedicine, especially in the individualized West, has been slow to adopt this terminology.

However, the concepts and tools of population health have been with us since the beginning of the twentieth century when biomedicine accepted an international classification of diseases, a tool that has most use when studying diseases in populations. Sanger and Stopes, with their eugenic orientation, were clearly concerned about the reproductive health of populations. And both vaccines and screening tests such as the Pap smear are intended not just for individuals, but for entire populations. We may not often call it "population health," but we have been practicing it for a century.

Control

Now, in order to effectively manage people with chronic diseases, practitioners need to ensure that patients regularly take their medicines and modify their diets and exercise patterns. And in order to effectively address the health problems of entire populations, biomedicine needs ways of effectively involving large numbers of people in its schemes: participating in screening, receiving vaccines, and changing behavior patterns. These tasks are far more complicated than simply giving a patient general anesthesia for an operation. Using anesthesia, the practitioner takes complete control of the unconscious patient, though for a very brief time. But effective chronic disease care and population health require patients who are awake and alert, and involved in their own care.

Ensuring this adherence to the medical regimen prescribed means that biomedicine must find methods of controlling people—yet without seeming to do so, because people do not like to be controlled. Consequently, as the century progressed, biomedicine saw the need for "health education" to properly inform people of their parts in chronic disease care and population health. The concept is optimistic: if people are properly educated, they will act differently. In fact, behavior change is never that easy, so biomedicine does what any technology does when it needs to control people's behavior: it engages the services of advertising[29] (now sometimes called "social marketing") and propaganda as we will see later. This is not to suggest that biomedicine lies about what it is offering. True propaganda, to be effective, must deal only in facts[30]— which is precisely what biomedicine does.

29. Packard, *Hidden Persuaders*.

30. Ellul, *Propaganda*, 53.

3

Medicalization: World War II to 1980

B Y THE MIDDLE OF the twentieth century, after the developed West had sorted out its destructive conflict with itself in two wars (occupying the same time period we have just finished examining), there were three overlapping currents occurring within biomedicine. All are consequences of the progress of the previous period and are clear mostly in retrospect. The first two help us put in perspective the third, medicalization, which is the subject of this chapter.

The first current is simply the continuation of the biotechnological advances we have just seen, only more complex and proceeding at a faster rate. Beginning in the 1940s chemotherapy was added to surgery and radiation as a promising method of treating cancer. In the early 1950s Watson and Crick discovered the structure of DNA, laying the foundation for today's remarkable progress in understanding genetics. By the mid 1950s we had a heart-lung machine and could do open heart surgery, and by 1960 chronic renal dialysis was available. The 1960s also brought us the first successful heart and liver transplantations, and the first kidney transplant from an unrelated donor.

All of these developments were dramatically effective in checking the progress of disease in an individual, if not always leading to a complete cure. Many of them addressed major life-threatening illnesses and successfully postponed what had not long before been sure death. Possibly the most emblematic of these developments were the Intensive Care Units (ICUs) of the early 1960s, and their community counterpart CPR (cardio-pulmonary resuscitation). CPR, though rarely successful in truly reversing cardio-pulmonary arrest, is very dramatic when it does.

ICUs, on the other hand, routinely maintain vital pulmonary, renal, and even cardiac functions in people who would certainly be dead without this maintenance. This "critical care" may have only a minor impact on the overall health of a population statistically, but its visibility—and its ability to mechanically prevent death—make it a social and ethical as well as a scientific phenomenon.

In fact, the ability to prolong biological life in people whose vital organs had failed put biomedicine in a difficult position: what to do next with the person being kept alive? Was discontinuing the mechanical life support equivalent to killing the person? The ability to postpone death brought into bold relief questions about the definition, and even the meaning, of life itself. It was in this context that bioethics expanded greatly at the end of this period, around 1980.

The second current is related to, and grows out of, the first. As biomedicine became more powerful, it became more risky to use, more dangerous.[1] The most obvious consequence of this danger is that the very technology intended to alleviate disease could end up causing other disease. This is iatrogenic (literally physician-caused) disease, a word Ivan Illich popularized in *Medical Nemesis* in 1976. Though his presentation of the problem was intentionally provocative at the time—his first sentence was "The medical establishment has become a major threat to health"[2]—parts of his critique have today become mainstream. By the end of the twentieth century (though already deeply into our third historical period), the Institute of Medicine in the US published *To Err Is Human: Building a Safer Health System*, suggesting that between 44,000 and 98,000 Americans die every year because of medical errors.[3] But these are just deaths from *errors*. If non-error iatrogenic disease is added in—that is, diseases doctors unintentionally cause, often from side effects of their medicines and technology—the numbers are two to three times higher.[4]

This disease-producing "side effect" of biotechnology naturally takes away from some of the benefits of that same biotechnology. As we have seen, Illich called those benefits *productivity*, and the negative side

1. Beck, *Risk Society*, ". . . the sources of wealth are 'polluted' by growing 'hazardous side effects.'" (20).

2. Illich, *Medical Nemesis*, 3.

3. Kohn et al., *To Err Is Human*.

4. Starfield, "Is US Health Really the Best?" 483–85.

effects *counterproductivity*.[5] These two stages correspond with our first two time periods: productivity, our first period, followed by counterproductivity, the post-World War II period. For Illich, however, counterproductivity wasn't just damage or "error"; it was actual reduction and even reversal of the stated goals of whatever technology was being considered. Schools, he claimed, kept us from learning; mechanical transport slowed us down.

To fully understand this health-denying or disease-producing effect of modern biomedicine—of biohealth itself—we need to examine medicalization, the third current. As we begin, it is important that we clarify exactly what medicalization is, and not demonize it. To medicalize something is simply to bring it under the realm and authority of biomedicine. If I have pain in the right lower part of my abdomen that has been there for a day or so, and I have a fever and no appetite, it would be very sensible for me to "medicalize" this pain: there is a good chance I have appendicitis. If on the other hand I get a pain in the right lower part of my abdomen every Christmas—and remember on reflection that it was around Christmas several years previously that a close relative died unexpectedly from complications of appendicitis—then it does not help for me to medicalize my pain. It may be more sensible to "psychologize" it. Medicalization is not by definition a value judgment; it is simply a description.

Admittedly the term "medicalization" is usually used in the sense of *inappropriate* medicalization; that is the sense that Illich used, that contemporary scholars use, and that I will be using. Nevertheless, the best way to see inappropriate medicalization is to see it in the context of appropriate medicalization, with which it is often in dynamic tension. That should become clear in the five examples that follow. I have chosen these five as paradigmatic of the process of medicalization before 1980, though some were medicalized even during the first pre-war period, and their medicalizing continues unabated into the current period of biohealth.

5. Illich, *Conviviality*, 1–9.

CHILDBIRTH—MEDICALIZING NORMALITY

Childbirth provides an excellent beginning for a discussion of medicalization for several reasons. It nicely illustrates the dynamic tension between appropriate and inappropriate medicalization, and it began so long ago that we can not only see it in perspective, but we can also see the demedicalizing backlash beginning during this post-war period. The medicalizing itself, however, began even before our first period, in the middle of the nineteenth century.

The pivotal year was 1848. In that year, in Vienna, Austria, Dr. I. F. Semmelweis published his findings of the benefits of doctors washing their hands before delivering babies. The previous year he had noted a marked difference in puerperal fever among women delivered in the hospital by midwives (2 percent) compared with those delivered by doctors (13 percent). When he simply mandated hand washing by the doctors (who often came straight from the autopsy room to the delivery room), the infection rate among the women delivered by doctors fell to almost the same as the midwife-delivered rate. He was, however, ostracized by Vienna doctors for implying that doctors were the reason for puerperal fever, and eventually left the city. After he left, hand washing stopped, and the puerperal fever rate among women delivered by doctors went back up—to nearly 20 percent.[6]

In the same year, 1848, Dr. Walter Channing in Boston published his findings of the use of ether anesthesia during delivery. He had first used this new development the year before for a difficult instrumental delivery of a dead fetus, with a very good outcome for the mother. However, he was not the first to use anesthesia for childbirth. A month before, Fanny Appleton Longfellow, the wife of Henry Wadsworth Longfellow, decided she wanted to try ether for her own normal delivery. She summoned a dentist—ether was first used as dental anesthesia in 1846 in Boston, and the Longfellows lived across the river in Cambridge—and had a successful home delivery by a midwife while the dentist administered ether to Fanny.[7]

These two stories appear at first to be examples of appropriate medicalization. Despite their inauspicious beginning, aseptic deliveries by doctors became commonplace and as a result puerperal fever was even-

6. Seri, "Historical Perspectives," e235–e238.
7. Kass, "My brother preaches, I practice."

tually controlled. And the need for adequate anesthesia for instrumental deliveries, and ultimately caesarean sections, is obvious. However, the story does not end there.

Even though both Semmelweis and Channing did their studies in hospitals, by 1900 most women still delivered at home—in the US, over 95 percent. Beginning about then, some women began to choose hospital deliveries, because that is where they could have a "painless birth" with anesthesia. By 1921, a third to a half of US women were delivering in hospitals. Also by this time, however, another factor had entered. In 1915 Dr. Joseph DeLee in Chicago published a paper claiming that childbirth was equivalent to a pathological process, and in 1920 proposed that every woman in labor be sedated, be given anesthesia during the second stage, be given an episiotomy, and have her baby delivered by forceps. (As much as I can determine, that is the way I was delivered in 1949.) All of this, of course, would also require a hospital delivery. By 1939, half to three-quarters of all US women delivered in hospitals; by 1950 85 percent, and by 1960 97 percent.[8]

Now the line between appropriate and inappropriate medicalization begins to get blurred. Giving birth is a normal, though admittedly sometimes dangerous, life event. Appropriate medicalization should treat the complications and if possible prevent the dangers; inappropriate medicalization treats every birth as a pathological process, or mandates that every birth come under the aegis of biomedicine. Let us look at historically how we have mixed the two.

Hand washing first. Using aseptic technique in assisting a woman to deliver is clearly important in preventing infection. But hand washing can hardly be seen as medicalization, and certainly does not require a hospital delivery. In 1848, before the germ theory of disease was at the foundation of biomedicine, midwives were as unaware of the microbial cause of puerperal fever as were doctors—yet the infection rate in their patients was low. Semmelweis's efforts only succeeded in bringing the infection rate of doctors' patients down to the level of midwives' patients. What he actually achieved was *demedicalization*: removing the iatrogenic effects of doctor-assisted deliveries. It was this demedicalizing that got him in trouble with the medical establishment.

Anesthesia next. Channing appropriately medicalized pain control and relaxation for difficult instrumental deliveries for obstructed labor.

8. Feldhusen, "History of Midwifery."

But Fanny Longfellow's first US use of anesthesia for childbirth was classic medicalization: the placing of a normal event under the authority and influence of biomedicine. The move toward hospital deliveries in the first half of the twentieth century was primarily a move toward "painless" childbirth, and only secondarily (under DeLee) a move toward "safer" childbirth.

Now DeLee. DeLee obviously recognized the risks inherent in childbirth, but—as is the case with all risk—it is difficult to determine which of those "at risk" will be affected. DeLee's approach was proactive: instead of waiting for problems to occur, he intervened in all women in labor, thereby gaining control of the process.[9] In a sense, he moved the risk from "out there" to "in here"; from the woman's home, where he could not see what was going on, to the hospital, where he could. But even more, he moved the risk from a natural process over which he had no control (labor and delivery) to a more mechanical process he could control (anesthetized assisted delivery). He did not eliminate risk, but he moved all women with risk under his control, treating them all as if something had already gone wrong. Very likely he discovered and corrected numerous problems that would otherwise have caused damage to the mother or her newborn child. But in the process he made every pregnant woman a patient dependent on medical intervention, completely medicalizing an event that throughout history had been (like hunting) a risky but still normal event.

With childbirth, all of this medicalizing occurred in our first historical period. Yet by this post-war period of medicalization, there were already signs of a backlash against this medicalization, and by the 1970s it was fashionable to talk of "natural childbirth." Many pointed to the experience in the Netherlands, where even today a third of deliveries are done at home by midwives, with excellent perinatal statistics. But medicalization is hard to reverse. A few decades after the backlash began, midwife-assisted deliveries in the US had *risen* to only 5.5 percent by the mid 90s—most still in birth centers or hospitals—and the US cesarean section rate had *fallen* to 21 percent.[10] Today the backlash is dead: the US C-Section rate is now over 30 percent, with probably two-thirds of woman who deliver vaginally using epidural anesthesia.

9. Rooks, "Childbirth."

10. Feldhusen, "History of Midwifery."

We need to comment in conclusion about cesarean sections, because the C-section rate illustrates so well the distinction between appropriate and inappropriate medicalization. The UN publishes statistics of C-section rates in many countries, and also tabulates national maternal mortality rates—the number of women dying as a result of childbirth per 100,000 live births.[11] If every C-section were "necessary," then there would clearly be a correlation between C-sections and mortality: the higher the C-section rate, the lower the maternal mortality (MM). This is true for those countries with very high MMs (sometimes over 1000); they often have very low C-section rates—1–2 percent. However, higher C-section rates do not always bring the lowest MM. For example, Dominican Republic has a C-section rate of 31 percent, and an MM of 150; Portugal has about the same rate (30 percent), but an MM of only 11. On the other hand, the Czech rate is only 14 percent, but still with a quite low MM—4. Yet Bolivia, with almost the same C-section rate (15 percent) has a MM of 290.

The "tipping point" seems to be a C-section rate of about 10 percent: Switzerland's rate is that, with an MM of only 5 (though Viet Nam's rate is the same, with an MM of 150). But below a 10 percent C-section rate, almost all countries have MMs significantly above 100. The point is clear: a national C-section rate of around 10 percent or a bit more might represent appropriate medicalization of birthing; a rate beyond about 15 percent probably represents inappropriate medicalization.

One final point about infant mortality: could it be that a high C-section rate will lower infant mortality (IM)? It's an intriguing idea, as all of the countries with low IMs (less than 10 infant deaths per 1,000 live births) have C-Section rates above 10 percent. However, the picture is the same as with MM—much higher C-Section rates do not lower infant mortality. Portugal and Switzerland both have IMs of about 4, with vastly different C-Section rates. In fact, it is not medicalization that lowers infant mortality, but economics.

ALCOHOLISM—MEDICALIZING SUBSTANCE ABUSE

Humans have always had a penchant for overusing or abusing some of the fruits of our post-Eden garden. Not all of them: not usually onions or

11. World Health Organization, Statistical Information System.

pencils or socks or songs or sleep, but certainly fermented fruit (alcohol) and opium and food and sex and games (such as gambling), and more recently beef and electronic entertainment. We regard some of these abuses as clearly wrong—sinful or illegal or both—especially abuse of each other and forced sex. But for the rest, while most societies frown on these excesses, we have no clear agreement on what sort of "wrong" they are. In some times and places we have spiritualized these abuses, making them sins. Or we have legalized (or really "illegalized") them, making them crimes. More recently, especially under the regimes of biomedicine and biohealth, we have medicalized many of these abuses: now they are diseases.

The idea that deviant behaviors such as these could be diseases dates to at least a century before our first period of biomedicine. Dr. Benjamin Rush, a signer of the US Declaration of Independence, developed an extensive theory of deviant behavior and social problems being diseases, including not only alcohol abuse but even lying.[12] Though this theory did not immediately become widely accepted, it kept being reintroduced by doctors and other influential people throughout the nineteenth century.[13] However, for several reasons during the first half of the twentieth century the disease idea almost disappeared:[14] the US pursed a completely legal approach to alcohol abuse, amending their constitution in 1919 to make the manufacture and sale of "intoxicating liquors" illegal. Prohibition was the antithesis of medicalization.

However, following Prohibition (the constitutional amendment was repealed fourteen years later), two developments occurred to strengthen the disease theory.[15] The first was the birth in 1935 of Alcoholics Anonymous. This self-help movement consisting of Twelve Steps was rooted in the idea that alcoholism was due to a physical reaction some people had to alcohol, much like an allergy. To AA, alcoholism was a disease; the therapy was alcoholics helping each other to follow the Twelve Steps, which involved voluntarily avoiding alcohol completely. However, AA did not use a *biomedical* therapy and has never been under the control of the medical system. It helped medicalize alcoholism, but did not medicalize its treatment.

12. Szasz, *Theology of Medicine*, 124.

13. White, "Addiction as a Disease," 46–51, 73.

14. White, "Rebirth of the Disease Concept," 62–66.

15. Schneider, "Deviant Drinking," 361–372.

The second development was the opening of the Yale Center for Alcohol studies, shortly before World War II. One of the principal researchers there, and its first director, was E. M. Jellinek, who published much of his work on alcoholism in the post-war period. His most widely quoted research was an analysis of some selected questionnaires given to members of AA. Based on these findings, Jellinek proposed several stages of progression in the disease of alcoholism, as well as several types of alcoholism. These observational studies and their biomedical language gave a boost to the growing post-war medicalization of all disease, and in 1956 the AMA said that the medical profession "recognizes this syndrome of alcoholism as an illness . . ."[16]

Alcoholism—that is, overuse of alcohol apparently beyond the control of the user, leading to harm of the self and others—seems to be a real entity and clearly remains a problem in most societies. Interestingly, how to classify it (a disease? a social problem? a moral shortcoming?) remains a matter of debate, even today. Contemporary critiques of a pure disease model, in fact, point to some of the problems with any medicalization.

For example, in a recent book review of *Biomedicalization of Alcohol Studies*, the reviewer summarized the central contention of the book thusly: "an emphasis on the individual biological and genetic determinants of 'alcoholism' will distract us from attending to the social consequences of alcohol use and undermine population-level strategies for reducing alcohol-related harm."[17] On the other hand, critics writing from a moral perspective have a different problem with medicalization: "The disease concept strips the substance abuser of responsibility."[18] In other words, for sociologists, medicalization takes away social responsibility; for moralists, medicalization takes away personal responsibility.

At first glance it appears that the characterization of alcoholism as a disease is shaky, at least historically. Despite the encouragement of Rush and others in the nineteenth century, the disease concept did not become established then, and seemed absent at the beginning of the twentieth century. Even now the debate is not over, with substantive social and moral critiques of medicalization. How then does biohealth, built solidly on medicalization, characterize alcoholism?

16. Schneider, "Deviant Drinking," 368.

17. Hall, "Biomedicalization of Alcohol Studies," 494–95.

18. Baldwin Research Institute, "Alcoholism."

Once again, as we saw in the last chapter, biohealth is not concerned with values or with meaning; it is concerned with scientifically verifiable evidence, and with control. Biohealth does not enter the discussion of whether or not a problem involving people is a disease. It simply assumes that any problem affecting human health is ultimately biological (hence the term bio-health), and consequently subject to control. That control is now mostly biological control, effected by medicines and surgery.

However, the desire to control biological phenomena is older than our ability to do so biologically, resulting initially in some draconian measures. We previously looked at eugenics in the early twentieth century: the desire to enable everyone to have a good birth by improving the gene pool of the race or nation—accomplished in those days by forced sterilizations, fully legal then in half the states of the US. Prohibition occurred during the very same time: an attempt to control the problem of alcohol abuse by a national law. Biohealth would repudiate these methods but not the control that underlies them. Biohealth does not care whether people call a problem "a disease"; its only concern is that biohealth experts (doctors, nurses, counselors, therapists) using biological methods diagnose, treat, or manage the problem. This will become clear in the section on medicalizing differences in appearance.

ADHD, CFS, AND SOCIAL PHOBIA—MEDICALIZING DEVIANCE

While alcoholism is a substance abuse, it is also a deviant behavior, deviating from the social norm of being able to control alcohol intake. There are many other deviant behaviors that do not involve substance abuse, but that we have medicalized—more recently, however, than alcoholism. It may be that they only became medicalized when we medicalized so many other areas of our lives in this period. It may also be that these behavior patterns did not previously exist, and now when we identify a new pattern, we put a medical label on it. Here we will look briefly at three of them.

Hyperactivity, especially in children, has been recognized by medicine for over a century. Not surprisingly, it was thought initially (1902) by some to be a "defect of moral control."[19] By the 1960s it had been medicalized: it was called "minimal brain dysfunction," and psycho-

19. Eli Lilly, "ADHD Timeline."

stimulants were used to treat it. By 1968 it was included in the official Diagnostic and Statistical Manual of Mental Disorders, second edition (DSM-II), and was then called "hyperkinetic reaction of childhood." Now we call it ADHD—attention deficit hyperactivity disorder.

As the name implies, ADHD is a behavior pattern of children who cannot focus their attention on something to the same extent as their peers and who are impulsive and overactive. Their behavior deviates from the norm of their classmates—or is it from the norm established by the classroom?—and is therefore deviant. But do they deviate from the norm because there is something wrong in their bodies—a disease—or do they deviate because they have learned or been taught to? Or could there even be, for some children, something deviant about the norm established by the classroom?[20] If studies uncover abnormal neuro-chemical or imaging or brain wave findings, are these the cause of the abnormal behavior, or the result? And if medication "normalizes" these abnormalities temporarily, does that prove the disease theory?

Some of these same sorts of questions have been raised by scholars about the second condition, chronic fatigue syndrome (CFS). While this condition did not apparently exist before the 1980s, it is possible that what had previously been called "neurasthenia" is essentially the same thing.[21] Now, however, we can do far more extensive testing than in the nineteenth century when the diagnosis of neurasthenia was popular—and now we find no consistent evidence of infectious or metabolic disorders with CFS. But we certainly find people who are chronically fatigued and who cannot work as a result. Do they have a disease—or more specifically, a biomedical disease?

One scholar, reviewing the medical literature on CFS in Israel, notes that although many etiologies have been considered, "the social etiology has been completely excluded, as has the possibility that this 'syndrome' is not a disease but an existential condition associated with certain forms of social organization."[22] In other words, could it be that some people are terribly tired as a response to the hectic life of the industrial world? Or is their fatigue a mirror of that tired world? In fact, could some children with ADHD or some adults with CFS be metaphorically responding to the pressures in the world in which they

20. Graham, "Politics of ADHD."
21. Meridian Institute, "Chronic Fatigue Syndrome and Neurasthenia."
22. File, "Medical Text," 1279.

find themselves? There is a similar argument for anorexia nervosa, that it "articulates contradictory and ultimately harmful cultural expectations of women."[23] In the same way that prophets proclaim and artists perform responses to our world in symbolic ways, could these sensitive people be responding with their bodies to "certain forms of social organization" that they find intolerable? These questions are unlikely to be formulated by biomedical science because they cannot be answered with randomized controlled trials.

Finally, social phobia. Shyness—or as some may prefer to call it, pathological shyness—was first considered a problem by some psychiatrists in the early twentieth century, but did not get official recognition as a disease (called "social fears") until the second edition of the DSM in 1968. Subsequent editions have kept the concept but changed the name; in the DSM-III (1980) it was "social phobia," and in the DSM-IV (1994) it was "social anxiety disorder (SAD)." About this time, three new psychotropic drugs were approved by the FDA for the treatment of SAD.[24]

Just as it is clear that some children are hyperactive and some adults are chronically tired, so it is clear that some people are shyer than others. Some are very shy. What is less clear is whether these behavior patterns that deviate from their surrounding norms are in fact diseases, or responses to social situations, as suggested above. The importance of this distinction is in determining whether medications are the most appropriate approach. However, teasing out these questions becomes very difficult when shy people hear (from pharmaceutical company advertising) that there are drugs to "treat" what they hadn't even realized was a "disease." In fact, pharmaceutical companies sometimes market diseases as aggressively as they market drugs.[25]

With these examples, the medicalizing emperor begins to look threadbare, if not naked. Bearing children can and does kill women; addictions seem, like many diseases, to be outside of a person's control. There is a valid debate here about appropriate and inappropriate medicalization. And yes, some few people are profoundly hyperactive, are disabled by extreme fatigue, or are pathologically aversive to social interaction. But calling fidgety or tired or shy people sick requires some mental gymnastics—more so, even, than seeing their behaviors as re-

23. Morris, *Illness and Culture*, 155.

24. About.com, "Social Anxiety Disorder."

25. Moynihan et al., "Selling Sickness," 886–91.

flections of modern industrial society. We will return to this at the end of this chapter.

COSMETIC SURGERY—MEDICALIZING APPEARANCE

The first two examples of medicalization clearly began long before this second time period we have characterized as "Medicalization"; some of the examples we just considered extend far into the present period. Cosmetic surgery, however, is a classic example of rapid development in the post-war period, and shows how medical influence can spread far beyond disease.

Cosmetic surgery is part of the larger field of Plastic Surgery, which involves reconstructive procedures as well as cosmetic ones. Reconstructive procedures repair scarred wounds or congenital defects; cosmetic procedures remove wrinkles, change nose shape, or make breasts larger or smaller. This desire to change appearance dates to long before even the modern medical period. There is evidence that surgeons in the ancient world attempted cosmetic alterations of facial injuries.[26] Francis Bacon, one of the fathers of Renaissance-era science, published a scientific utopia called *New Atlantis* in 1627, and at the end he appended a list of achievements he foresaw science offering for the "benefit of mankind." Among them were "The restitution of youth in some degree," "The altering of complexions, and fatness and leanness," and "The altering of features."[27] The roots of modern plastic surgery date to the origins of modern science.

However, only recently have surgeons successfully "altered complexions and features." The medical advances of the nineteenth century that enabled surgery to flourish—anesthesia, infection control, and increased understanding of anatomy and physiology—were the foundations on which the surgeons of the First World War developed effective techniques for reconstructing facial war wounds. Technically, the same skills necessary to rebuild a face destroyed by shrapnel could also be used to remodel a face according to the dictates of beauty or fashion. Yet using surgery for "disease" is far from using it for "desire." The gap needed to be addressed, and plastic surgeon Max Thorek addressed it:

26. Backstein and Hinek, "War and Medicine," 217–19.
27. Bacon, *New Atlantis* 185–86.

"If soldiers whose faces had been torn away by bursting shell on the bat-
tlefield could come back into an almost normal life with new faces created by the wizardry of the new science of plastic surgery, why couldn't
women whose faces had been ravaged by nothing more explosive than
the hand of the years find again the firm clear contours of youth?" There
was "no stranger aftermath" of that war, he suggested, "than the sudden
hope, surging through feminine—and sometimes masculine—hearts,
that where nature had been niggardly in her gifts of pulchritude, the
knife of the surgeon could remedy the lack."[28]

Advances from the First World War created the possibilities, but it
wasn't until after the Second World War that cosmetic surgery rapidly
developed, especially with successful breast implants and liposuction.[29]
Nevertheless, the field of plastic surgery was still predominantly reconstructive rather than cosmetic in this post-war period, and remained
that way—until this century. Only in 2000, according to the American
Society of Plastic Surgeons, did the number of cosmetic procedures
done by their members begin to exceed the number of reconstructive
procedures.[30] Medicalization began in the post-war period, but it certainly did not end then.

Max Thorek's statement is a ringing endorsement, not simply of
cosmetic surgery, but of this entire concept of medicalization. With
Thorek, medical technique does not slyly sneak in the back door of areas
of our lives unused to it; rather it opens the front door and boldly an-
nounces itself. Why not change our appearance if we want to, and can
do so successfully? There is no doubt here that "the hand of the years"
is anything but negative, that "nature" can truly be "niggardly." There is
even none of the usual recourse to the negative psychological effects of
teasing and shame from disfigured features, making treatment of them
a medical necessity. This is a naked celebration of the medicalization of
appearance. But more than this, it introduces us to the idea that humans
cannot merely be made *different* by science, they can be made *better*. We
now call this "human enhancement."

Human enhancement, if not an oxymoron, is at least a startling
concept—now actively being pursued by genetic engineering. Enhance

28. Quoted in Haiken, *Venus Envy,* chapter 1.

29. Tackla, "Phoenix from the Flames."

30. American Society of Plastic Surgeons, "Media—Statistics."

means "to increase in value, quality, desirability, or attractiveness."[31] Can we really increase the value of a human by biomedical means? It appears that we *can* increase the attractiveness or desirability of people, but those are qualities "in the eye of the beholder"—not inherent human value. The ethical question underneath this is, "*Should* we change humans?"— a question worth debating.[32] But the deeper question is really, "*Can* we fundamentally change humans?" Is there a eugenic human alchemy whereby we can truly improve the inherent value of humans?

In our world saturated by images, we can easily get confused between appearance and reality—or we can consciously equate appearance with reality. We can also of course affirm the difference, and when we do we begin to see the starkness of the question: Does anything biomedicine does really enhance, or improve the inherent value of, humans?

Finally, before leaving cosmetic surgery, we need to look briefly at how this form of medicalization can become counterproductive. Often the rationale given for changing someone's appearance is their psychological distress, either from being teased or from their own inner sense of shame or inadequacy. But apparently pre-operative evaluation of that psychological distress is imperfect. A large recent study of women who had received cosmetic breast implants in Sweden showed they had a three-fold increase in deaths from suicide and alcohol or drug dependence, as well as excess deaths from accidents and injuries. Admittedly this excess may not be a result of the implants themselves, but rather a reflection of some "underlying psychiatric morbidity" that may have previously manifested itself in dissatisfaction with their breast size.[33] Nevertheless, the question remains: Was the implant procedure productive or counterproductive?

SCREENING—MEDICALIZING PREVENTION

To prevent is to keep from happening. That is certainly a noble goal when it comes to disease. It is also rarely a medical matter. People do not generally *develop* diseases because they lack medicine or surgery.

31. Merriam-Webster's 11th Collegiate Dictionary.

32. Little, "Cosmetic Surgery," 162ff.

33. Lipworth, "Excess Mortality among Women with Cosmetic Breast Implants," 119–23.

They develop diseases because they inherited them, or because of environmental toxins or carcinogens, or because a microbe entered their body from contaminated air or food or water or from another person, or because they move and eat in ways their bodies weren't evolved (or designed) for, or because of stress, or because of injury. Or for reasons we haven't figured out yet. This is obvious.

However, as our knowledge of diseases expanded early in the twentieth century, medical science began to recognize early forms of disease, not evident to the "patient," but discoverable by careful questioning or by laboratory tests. Discovering these early forms of disease was not true prevention, but very often these early forms could be successfully managed or even cured. Public health reflects this new form of prevention in their terminology: while *primary* prevention is keeping the disease from happening in the first place, *secondary* prevention is finding the disease in an early or pre-symptomatic form (i.e., screening) and providing treatment while it is still beneficial.

Or, to use the terminology of this chapter, secondary prevention is medicalized prevention (though not necessarily inappropriate medicalization). Another term suggested is "surveillance medicine,"[34] constantly watching and examining a healthy population for early signs of disease. Surveillance medicine began in the early years of the twentieth century, focusing especially on children in the UK to ensure that their development was according to the norms then being developed. Another early use of surveillance was screening American military recruits in World War I for psychiatric disease.[35] In both of these early examples, there were very discrete populations being screened.

However, as we move into this period of medicalization, the surveillance becomes more widespread. As our understanding of diseases and ability to detect them early both improved, we have added other conditions we screen for, as well as expanded our vista for surveillance. For a half dozen or so conditions today, most adherents to biomedicine advocate for screening the *entire* population. And the roots of all of these screening programs are in this period of medicalization.

We have already looked at the development of the Pap smear to screen for cervical cancer. Though the technology for screening was available at the end of the first period, it is mostly in the post-war period

34. Armstrong, "Rise of Surveillance Medicine," 395.
35. Morabia and Zhang, "History of Medical Screening," 463–69.

that Pap smear screening developed *as a program*. And, as a program, we recommend screening for *all* women, regardless of "risk factors." The second widely recommended screening program today is mammography for breast cancer, and the first modern instrument for taking mammograms was developed in the early 1950s. However, it was only in the 1960s that it became an acceptable technology for widespread screening—and again, the recommendation is for *all* women beyond a certain age.

Also in the early 1960s epidemiological research demonstrated very clear links between elevated cholesterol levels and heart disease, and likewise between elevated blood pressure and both heart disease and strokes. These then became the third and fourth conditions for which we recommend screening *all* people, both male and female, again regardless of risk factors.

By the late 1960s the connection between small amounts of blood in the stool and colon cancer was demonstrated, and colonoscopy became more widely available to confirm suspected cases of colon cancer. Fecal occult blood testing (and later, sigmoidoscopy or even colonoscopy) became the fifth screening procedure recommended for *everyone* beyond a certain age. And finally, at the end of our period in 1980, the PSA (prostate specific antigen) test was developed and introduced as a screening test for prostate cancer. Though more controversial than most of the others, for many biomedical practitioners this is the sixth screening procedure recommended for *all* men beyond a certain age.

Looking at these contemporary screening programs together provides us with an excellent final example of this period of medicalization, and begins pointing to what happens to a medicalized society as a result. Here it is important to repeat what we said earlier: medicalization is a descriptive term, not necessarily a critique. Studies show conclusively that some of these screening programs can reduce the incidence of disease and mortality in the population screened. We are not arguing that medicalization doesn't "work." Maternal mortality falls with medicalization, hyperactive children are calmer when they take psycho-stimulants, cosmetic surgery can remove wrinkles and modify breast size.

There are other questions besides effectiveness, however. Let's look again at these half-dozen screening programs. They are all examples of secondary prevention. Do we have corresponding *primary* prevention knowledge for these six? With two of them, we do not: we are not sure what women can *do* or *not do* to prevent breast cancer from occurring in the first place. Likewise we do not know what men can *do* to prevent prostate cancer from developing.

However, with the other four, there are known primary preventive activities. Cervical cancer has been linked to HPV (human papilloma virus), a sexually acquired infection; changing sexual behavior can prevent acquiring sexually transmitted diseases. Both colon cancer and high serum cholesterol are related to life-long diet, especially diets low in fiber and high in animal fat. And many, though not all, people with hypertension have "modifiable factors"—that is, salt intake, obesity, and stress.

None of these are secret observations, nor are they of minor importance. Celibate nuns do not get cervical cancer; Africans eating traditional diets rarely get colon cancer or coronary heart disease. These conditions truly are preventable—yet the preventions involved are not "medical." And in our medicalized society, "medical" testing and interventions are more trusted than "behavior change"—or really, "society change." While the need to change behavior or society does not mitigate against the use of screening tests, we must remember that screening tests will never change behavior or society.

And one final irony: the two conditions that we really don't know (yet?) how to prevent (breast and prostate cancer) have the most debatable screening programs with the least obvious results. Consequently, the studies to "prove" their minimal effectiveness need to be far larger and more complicated.[36]

SUMMARY

Now let's reflect on these five examples together to look more closely at what medicalization does to a society. Considering the very powerful and effective biomedical techniques developed during the twentieth century, it is understandable that we would begin assuming that these sorts of techniques should be used for every dis-ease. Unfortunately their effectiveness in general leads us to offer and use them even where we don't need to, where they displace adequate preexisting ways of doing the same thing—or, strangely, even when there is no dis-ease. The result

36. Morabia and Zhang, "History of Medical Screening," 463–69.

is that biomedicine grows in importance and authority in our societies, displacing or incorporating some of the functions that religion and law used to have.[37] In a medicalized society, biomedicine claims jurisdiction not only over disease, but also over unhappiness (such as shyness) and deviance (such as hyperactivity or alcoholism). It subsumes normal life events such as eating and exercise, birth and death, and even claims authority in aesthetics, as in cosmetic surgery. Biomedicine, originally intended to manage disease, now claims expertise even over its opposite, health, and allows medicalized prevention to upstage behavioral and social prevention, as we saw with screening.

There are at least three questions that grow out of the observation that biomedicine now has hegemony in our societies: Who controls it? What happens to our understanding of disease causation when biomedicine has hegemony? and What are the effects in society?

Control

By the 1970s scholars especially in the social sciences had recognized the process of medicalization, and proposed that a chief reason was control by medical professionals, especially doctors.[38] Indeed, in the early post-war period, medicalization did benefit doctors, giving them more business and money. But is medicalization fundamentally about control by doctors?

One optimistic view is that it was, and that centralized doctor control is now thankfully in retreat: "in the modern Internet information age [says one social scientist] medical knowledge has helped undermine medical authority and has encouraged individuals to take more responsibility for their own health care. My mother-in-law often knows more about the contraindications of the drugs her doctor prescribes than he does himself. When medical knowledge has been more widely circulated it has usually served individual rather than state interest."[39] While it is true that doctor control may be in retreat, medicalization is certainly not. When people get medical information from the Internet, that does not "undermine medical authority"; it is rather evidence of the hegemony of biomedical authority. The only thing undermined is

37. Zola, "Medicine as an Institution of Social Control," 487–504; and Zola "Healthism and Disabling Medicalization," 41–67.

38. Conrad, "Shifting Engines of Medicalization," 3–14.

39. Nye, "Evolution of the Concept of Medicalization," 115–29.

doctors' authority. Individuals in our societies have in fact internalized a biomedical view of life, albeit reinforced by doctors.

Another view is that while control of medicalization has shifted away from doctors, the shift has not been to individuals themselves, but to "commercial and market interests."[40] Indeed, there is always a close relationship between what people "want" and what commercial interests promote (or advertise). That individuals themselves obtain biomedical information from the Internet may "democratize" the availability of this information, but does nothing to challenge the need or appropriateness of this information—that is, to challenge medicalization. The market indeed has plenty of reasons to promote medicalization; a medicalized life is a life dependent on biomedical commodities.

Both of these views, taken together, give us an excellent preview of some characteristics of biohealth: information, individual responsibility, and market interests. We will discuss these more fully in Part II.

Disease Causation

When we medicalize all dis-ease, that means we accept the biomedical approach for understanding and managing diseases. Biomedicine always looks for a physical (genetic, infectious, toxic, etc) or psychological cause. Though medical analysis often comments on the "epidemiology" of a disease process, which may include social factors, it rarely attributes the fundamental cause to these social factors, as we saw with Chronic Fatigue Syndrome. The principle critique of medicalization by social scientists is that it "desocializes" disease,[41] that it ignores social factors in the etiologies of diseases, and consequently in their management.

This is not a new concept. Long before medicalization had begun— in fact even before our first period of biomedical developments—Rudolf Virchow was promoting a social view of disease. He saw the need to know the social conditions in which people lived, to see how these conditions affected people's health, and to intervene in these conditions to improve health.[42] To him, "Medicine is a social science, and politics nothing but medicine on a grand scale."[43] This view was upstaged by the

---

40. Conrad, "Shifting Engines of Medicalization," Abstract.

41. Filc, "Medical Text," 1275–85.

42. Rosen, *History of Public Health*, 230.

43. Quoted in Lander, *Defective Medicine*, 81.

dramatic biomedical advances of the late nineteenth and early twentieth centuries, but did not fully disappear. As we saw above, the period of alcohol Prohibition in the US attempted to intervene legally with one of the factors that affected health—and as such was the opposite of medicalization.

In the 1970s—during the growth of medicalization we have just documented—there was a renewal of a broader view of health, and the UN's Alma Ata conference on Primary Health Care in 1978 espoused a concept of health and disease far beyond the biomedical. But over the next two decades this broader "horizontal" approach came in conflict with disease-specific "vertical" programs in developing countries, and horizontal social approaches receded. However, some are attempting to resurrect this social approach on the thirtieth anniversary of Alma Ata: "The focus of the global health community," said a *Lancet* editorial in 2008, "is shifting from a biological to a social model of health, from vertical to horizontal programmes, and towards health-system strengthening."[44] And there is plenty of recent literature to support the notion that "health [should] become a social science."[45]

However, considering the very powerful commercial and market interests noted above, it will take far more that the "global health community" or the UN to reverse the process of medicalization.

Effects

Finally, we need to return to one of the observations we began this chapter with, that a medicalized world is a risky, dangerous world. But the risks are not simply from the powerful technologies themselves. Every medicalized society is also at risk of losing traditional religious and cultural ways of healing, ways that can never be replaced by biomedical methods. In *Medical Nemesis*, Illich devoted far more attention to what he called social and cultural iatrogenesis than he did to clinical iatrogenesis. These refer to what happens to a people when a technology, such as biomedicine, takes over the functions that previously were done by the community, family, or patient. The technology may actually be more effective or efficient in treating a particular illness, but Illich was asking what happened socially and culturally to communities when their previ-

44. Editorial in *The Lancet*, "Margaret Chan Puts Primary Health Care Centre Stage" 1811.

45. Wilkinson, *Unhealthy Societies*, chapter 2.

ous independence in matters of suffering and healing is transformed to dependence on the medical system. He considered that movement from independence to dependence, from intransitive healing ("I healed") to transitive healing ("the doctor healed me"),[46] to be another form of iatrogenesis: physician-caused disease not in the individual, but in the community, in the entire culture.

This social and cultural iatrogenesis is a theme that runs along the edge of all of the examples above. When the medical system controls childbirth—and eventually child-rearing—we lose the ability to bear children, both physically and metaphorically. When alcoholism is a disease, individual and social responsibility have less meaning. When fidgety, tired, and shy people are seen to be sick, they need a medical system instead of culturally proven rituals. When beauty is only external (and modifiable by surgery) we lose the understanding of inner beauty. When prevention is what the medical system does, the society forgets how to remain healthy. It is no surprise that despite measurable improvements in health status in medicalized societies, people nevertheless are more dissatisfied, have more symptoms, and report more disability.[47]

46. Illich, *Medical Nemesis*, 119 n. 255.

47. Barasky, "Paradox of Health," 414–18.

4

Biohealth: 1980 to Present

I<small>T SHOULD BE CLEAR</small> by now that we are concerned in this study not merely with new medical technologies as they affect diseases, but also with the effects of these technologies on our societies. We are interested in what sorts of things happen to us individually, socially, culturally, and morally as a result of new medical technologies, especially the sorts of influences and pressures that are unique to our age.

Consequently the generalizations at the end of chapter 2 are all new to the post-1900 world: the hegemony of science as the foundation for healing, the life-long management of chronic diseases, the inclusion of the entire population as the object of medical services, and the need for control of the patients and potential patients as a result. Likewise in chapter 3, the medicalization of all of society, which followed from these developments, is an even more recent phenomenon in history. The dramatic, apparently miraculous triumphs of modern medicine over disease have been accompanied by these other new developments that affect the way we live and move and have our being in society.

All of this was in place by 1980. But it was all there as "pieces," and not yet as biohealth. It was a period, in the US at least, of "disarray,"[1] of "crisis."[2] Admittedly this American "disarray" was, and still is, economic: rising costs and falling healthcare coverage, which are intimately related to the US lack (unique among industrialized countries) of national health insurance. But this was not the crisis Ivan Illich referred to in *Medical Nemesis;* to him the deeper crisis was that the medical estab-

1. Fox, *Power and Illness*, chapter 4.
2. Ehrenreich, "Introduction: The Cultural Crisis," 1.

lishment itself was becoming "a major threat to health"—a problem big enough for him to chronicle several "political countermeasures" that he hoped would lead to "the recovery of health."[3] History, however, took a different route, and instead of a recovery of health brought us biohealth. Twenty years after *Medical Nemesis*, Illich repudiated his hope for a recovery of health,[4] and seeing why will become clear in Part II.

However, 1980 did not feel like a crisis point or a watershed year at the time. I was then five years out of medical school, had completed training in the relatively new and now popular field of Family Medicine, and was enjoying practice in a rural Appalachian community in East Tennessee. My biggest concerns were not the nature of medical care (despite having recently read *Medical Nemesis*) but it's availability to underserved communities, which our county was. I was responding to the most visible "crisis" in American medicine, which was access. Medicine itself was of course changing, but it seemed like medicine was *always* changing; it did not feel then like we were on the verge of a new period.

When our family moved to Africa in 1985, we were unaware then that anything fundamental was changing in the nature of modern medicine. We returned to the US in 1996 to practice for a year, and again in 2001 for three more years. It was during these visits that we began to realize something *was* changing in biomedicine. In 1996 the most obvious changes in the US were economic, with the new prominence of "managed care." However, in comparing the medicine we had been practicing in Africa with the medicine we now saw in the US,[5] we had a glimpse of how biomedicine itself was changing. But it was only a glimpse; it took another decade of reading and reflection for me to understand that something *did* happen around 1980, and that the practice of biomedicine is now fundamentally different from what I was taught in medical school.

The changes were of course gradual. But, as in the first two periods, there were developments and events that heralded or symbolized or precipitated the changes of that period. And this time, the events are clustered within just a few years of 1980.

---

3. Illich, *Medical Nemesis*, 3, chapters 7 and 8.

4. Illich, "Pathogenesis, Immunity, and the Quality of Public Health."

5. Downing, *Suffering and Healing in America.*

KAREN QUINLAN 1976

In 1975, Karen Ann Quinlan, adopted as an infant by religious Catholic parents, turned twenty-one. Shortly after her birthday, she moved in with some roommates a few miles away from her parents. About that time she also went on a very strict diet for a few days, and then attended a party with some friends. After consuming some alcohol and other drugs, she felt dizzy and lay down. A short time later friends found her unconscious and not breathing. They attempted resuscitation, and had her brought to a hospital where she was admitted comatose and placed on a ventilator.

Doctors at the hospital, after repeated examinations and tests, decided that she was in a "persistent vegetative state" and would not wake up. They also felt that the ventilator was needed to keep her breathing. Based on this information, her parents asked the doctors to disconnect the ventilator. The hospital refused, and Mr. Quinlan took the case to court. The lower court in New Jersey sided with the hospital and the doctors. On appeal, however, the New Jersey Supreme Court sided with Mr. Quinlan. Just over a year after she lost consciousness, in May 1976, doctors turned off the ventilator. In an ironic twist, Karen did not die. She was continued on tube feedings, and finally nine years later died of pneumonia.

Since the Quinlan case, there have been numerous other similar situations with court cases testing other end-of-life situations; witness the Terri Schiavo case where the legal matter was the very tube feedings that kept Karen Quinlan alive for ten years. And before Karen Quinlan became famous, doctors and relatives were undoubtedly faced numerous times with severely brain-damaged people on ventilators. What made Karen Quinlan's medical care so pivotal was the publicity. For the first time the general public together with the medical community had to wrestle with the power of biomedicine to keep someone alive who had no chance of improvement, and who would not be alive without the biotechnology.

Certainly one result was that more such cases were litigated. But more important for biohealth was that the Karen Quinlan case opened the door for medical ethics to play a much larger role in medical care. When I finished Family Medicine training at the University of Tennessee in Knoxville in 1978, I had not had even one lecture in medical ethics; when my wife finished the same program in 1980, medical ethics lectures were a routine part of the curriculum—linked with one of the first graduate programs in the US in medical ethics.[6] We will look more closely at the role of medical ethics in chapter 9.

BIOPSYCHOSOCIAL MODEL 1977

The year after the Karen Quinlan case, *Science* published what eventually came to be seen as a landmark article: "The Need for a New Medical Model: A Challenge for Biomedicine."[7] The author, George Engel, was a psychiatrist working at the University of Rochester, a center for Family Medicine research as well; its reputation drew my application the year before. (I chose Knoxville instead because I wanted to work in Appalachia.) Engel's article proposed that biomedicine adopt a broader model for diagnosing and treating disease, a model he called the biopsychosocial model. What it proposed is in many ways apparent from the name, and it was a model Family Medicine and other primary care specialties rapidly adopted.

While Engel's thesis—that social and psychological factors can influence illness as much as biological factors—was partly just common sense, he included a section at the end of his article that in retrospect may be the most important part: he connected his biopsychosocial model with general systems theory. He was, in doing this, linking his approach to medicine with a parallel movement occurring within philosophy. Just two years after his article, Jean-François Lyotard published *The Postmodern Condition*, now generally accepted as the official beginning of postmodern thinking. So what is the connection between biopsychosocial medicine, general systems theory, and postmodernism?

"I define postmodern as incredulity toward metanarratives."[8] This brief definition from Lyotard's 1979 book points to a hallmark of postmodern thinking, the suspicion of metanarratives, or grand over-arching explanations of knowledge or experience. For over a century, as we have seen, medicine subscribed to such a metanarrative, the germ theory of disease—or more generally, the "doctrine of specific etiology."[9] What

---

6. Thomasma, "Early Bioethics," 5–6.

7. Engel, "Need for a New Medical Model," 129–36.

8. Lyotard, *Postmodern Condition*.

9. Lander, *Defective Medicine*, 79.

Engel was proposing is that diseases often had many factors involved in their etiologies, not just a single germ or metabolic dysfunction, and that to diagnose and treat accurately and fully we need to consider multiple factors—psychological and social as well as physical—as they interrelate.

And this is where systems thinking comes in. General systems theory articulates this interrelationship of elements as the essence of a system. This systems thinking is, in fact, a postmodern understanding of illness. The "convergences between biology and culture . . . signal the end of the machine age and perhaps the advent of systems theory as a dominant metaphor for illness."[10] We will examine the importance of this more closely in the next chapter, chapter 5.

REAGAN 1980

The economic world today is different from the post-WWII economic world, and US President Ronald Reagan, elected in 1980, has been both praised and blamed for this difference. The theory of tax cuts and government deregulation to stimulate economic growth was even named after him—Reaganomics. Was he the cause? Or just a symbol or herald, as so many of the other events and developments we've reviewed?

While the cause of the post-1980 world economic changes is admittedly important, even more to the point of this discussion is what those changes were in biomedicine. Perhaps the most obvious is the increasing profitability of the pharmaceutical industry.[11] During the 1970s, overall industry median profits stayed around 4 percent, while drug industry profits were just about double that. Then, beginning around 1980, the all-industry median profit began to fluctuate a bit more, between 2 percent and 6 percent. However, beginning about the same time, pharmaceutical industry profits began rising, albeit with some fluctuations, but still climbing to over 18 percent by the end of the century. Industry overall may not have benefited by the changes in the early 1980s, but the pharmaceutical industry certainly did.

So how does pharmaceutical profitability affect health care, and more specifically the development of biohealth? First, as pharmaceutical companies became more profitable, they began shifting priorities in what

10. Morris, *Illness and Culture*, 6.
11. Public Citizen Congress Watch, "2002 Drug Industry Profits," 12.

they were producing. "During the 1980s the number of large drug companies producing vaccines declined from twelve to four."[12] Vaccines, in biohealth, are for everyone, but not everyone can afford them. Therefore production is not always highly profitable—and has the additional risk of lawsuits when a vaccine given to *all* healthy people results in side effects in a few. Drug companies have increasingly preferred to develop and produce "feel-good drugs, such as Prozac and Viagra," that wealthy consumers want and can pay for.[13]

Second, accompanying this profitability, there was a marked increase in pharmaceutical company mergers beginning in the late 1980s. Pfizer is among the world's largest pharmaceutical corporations today; its size stems from merging with at least seven of its major competitors, including Parke-Davis, Warner-Lambert, Searle, Upjohn—and, in 2009, Wyeth. The story is the same for Sanofi-Aventis, now a combination of at least nine mostly European competitors; and for GlaxoSmithKline, which swallowed or merged with thirteen competitors. While merging does not always make employees happy, and jobs are sometimes lost, the rationale is that research and development become more productive.[14] However, it is certainly open to question how useful this research is and how many new drugs that improve health are developed.[15]

Because of their size and profitability—and the presence of their products in our lives—pharmaceutical companies are an understandable focus for our attention. However, underneath their influence in our understanding of health was a 1982 US Supreme Court decision that had nothing to do with drug companies. Nothing directly, that is; but the decision clarified what health is in the present realm of biohealth, and drug companies were undoubtedly delighted.

In 1975, The US Federal Trade Commission (FTC) began an administrative action against the American Medical Association (AMA). The AMA had until then declared that physician advertising was unethical; the FTC claimed that such a prohibition was a restraint of trade inconsistent with US anti-trust laws. Though the immediate target was this almost obscure ethical principle, the context of the case was not at

12. Rempel, *High Price for Abundant Living,* 92.

13. Ibid.

14. Koenig and Mezick, "Are Pharmaceutical Company Mergers Rational?"

15. Angell, *Truth About the Drug Companies.*

all obscure.[16] The US, facing rising health care costs in the 1970s, had two options: either attempt to control costs through budgeting and oversight, which was the choice of most other industrialized nations, or depend on market competition—which would imply the use of advertising. The AMA, on the other hand, had used their anti-advertising "ethical" stance to limit the growth of non-private practice models such as HMOs. The government's deregulation sentiment of the 1980s had already begun, and the AMA was generating resentment because of its perceived role in protecting the interests of a powerful and rich profession. The battle lines were drawn.

It was a protracted battle. In 1978, after an eight month trial, the administrative law judge sided with the FTC. The AMA appealed, and four years later the Supreme Court also sided with the FTC. Physician advertising, which for centuries had been unethical, was suddenly ethical.

This, of course, was only an American decision, but the decision grows from an understanding of biohealth that is international: health is a commodity, subject to market forces, and can therefore be advertised. The US Supreme Court did not create this understanding, it only recognized what by 1982 already existed. Something still bothers us about this, and the whole idea of advertising still generates debate—but we understand that the debate has been lost: the title of a recent article on physician advertising contained the words "selling out" and "lamenting."[17] We still want very much to believe that "patients are not consumers in search of a commodity," as the article claims, but biohealth proclaims exactly the opposite. Health now *is* a commodity—the subject of chapter 7.

PC 1981

The personal computer (PC) did not suddenly appear to the world in 1981; like all of these 1980s developments there was a process of development and refinement, a process that is still going on with computers. But there were distinct steps.[18] Large commercial computers had been available since the 1950s, and continued to get physically larger as they

16. Ameringer, "Organized Medicine on Trial," 445–71.

17. Tomycz, "Profession Selling Out," 26–28.

18. About.com, "History of Computers."

became more powerful. During my Family Medicine training in the mid 1970s, the research computer in use then filled an entire room. During that same time, smaller home computer kits were marketed mostly as hobby items.

However, 1981 brought two distinct events: in August, IBM introduced a home computer and called it a "PC." Then in October, Osborne Computers released the first portable "laptop" computer. Though that computer was bulky and not successful, it was the beginning of laptops. By December, *Time Magazine* saw the future of personal computers, and called the computer the "man of the year" for 1981.

As everywhere in the modern world, computers are ubiquitous in medicine. Anywhere machines are used in medicine, there is a likelihood that an advanced model has been developed utilizing computer technology—including "robot surgery" carried out in one city, with the surgeon controlling the robot located in a different city, operating over the internet. Diagnostic machines were early adopters of the computer: CAT (*computed* axial tomography) scans were introduced in the 1970s. And over the last decade, electronic medical records are becoming the standard of care, with clinicians typing the patient's story into the computer during the interview.

There are, however, two particular uses of computers that expanded in the 1980s; both play significant roles in biohealth. James Le Fanu suggests in *The Rise and Fall of Modern Medicine*[19] that a "new paradigm emerged quite dramatically in the 1980s driven by two very different specialties . . . : epidemiology and genetics." Both attempt to identify the underlying causes of disease—"nature (the gene) and nurture (social and environmental factors)"—and both incidentally rely heavily on computer technology. Le Fanu's view is that neither has been successful in improving our lives, and "the failure of the two great projects . . .—he New Genetics and The Social Theory [underpinned by epidemiology]—constitute the fall of modern medicine." Genes, he says, "do not play an important role in disease," and "the Social Theory has had near enough zero effect on the nation's health." These may be overstatements, but their corollaries are nevertheless true: focusing only on genetics is too reductionistic an approach to explain the major causes of ill health, and focusing only on behavior change as suggested by epidemiology's Social

19. Le Fanu, *Rise and Fall of Modern Medicine*, 239, 339.

Theory amounts to victim-blaming. We will examine further the wider notion of personal responsibility for health in chapter 8.

Biohealth, of course, does not agree that modern biomedicine has "fallen." In its inclusive way, it embraces both genetics and epidemiology despite their flaws. Or more accurately, it swallows both and ignores their flaws. Biohealth foresees the possibility of control, even if only partial, through gene change and behavior change—both, of course, voluntary.

But more than just swallowing and ignoring critiques such as Le Fanu's, biohealth bypasses them. Certainly the influence of genes in many diseases, and the health improvement brought about by behavior change, may be minimal. But these changes are often *statistically significant*, a term we now often use when an effect is so small that it is not clinically significant. And we can determine statistical significance from very large epidemiologic studies, so large and complicated that we need computers to analyze the results.

We are back to where we started in 1900 with the International Classification of Diseases (ICD), only now computers have enabled us to make much fuller use of its data. Computers also enable us to predict, based on huge amounts of data, what *might* happen to us, what our *risk* of a disease is. This hallmark of biohealth is the subject of chapter 6.

SUMMARY

We have introduced the major topics of Part II. But before leaving this idiosyncratic review of twentieth-century events that paved the way for biohealth, we need to look at one last characteristic of them: social class. Understandably, the biomedical advances mentioned in these three chapters originated in the scientific communities of Western and Westernized countries—often connected with medical establishments and universities, representing the elite of those countries. Nevertheless, the products of their research were intended for everyone, regardless of wealth or social class. Biomedicine, created by a rich Western elite, would like its products to be universal. Any diabetic in the world should get insulin, an alcoholic in any culture should be considered ill, birth control should be available to every woman.

The events in this chapter, on the other hand, are different. They are hallmark events not for *biomedical* advances, but for characteristics or elements of *biohealth*; not for the technology, but for how we use it. And these characteristics very much mirror the society in which they developed: a middle class, Western society.[20] Notions of systems, risk, personal responsibility for a sort of health that is a commodity—all of these ideas grow out of a particular culture and world view, and seem sensible or even obvious within that culture. But can they claim to be as universal as the offerings of biomedicine? The question has importance because biohealth, like biomedicine before it, is being exported all over the world. We will examine this more fully in Part III.

20. Crawford, "Health as a Meaningful Social Practice," 401–20.

PART II

The Elements of Biohealth

MEDICALIZATION WAS FAIRLY COMPLETE by 1980. We had brought (or in some cases begun to bring) all areas of life under the aegis of biomedicine. But biomedicine could not, of course, take care of everything; it could not adequately do what law, religion, education, and other parts of society had always done. If the development of biomedicine was being controlled by a company or a committee or a government, perhaps that committee or government could have recognized the inappropriate medicalizations and tried to control them.

But there is no such international committee. Biomedicine is part of what Jacques Ellul called the technological society: the world-wide growth, and ultimately hegemony, of technology in our lives, especially since World War II.[1] Of course modern medical technologies began centuries ago, as we saw in Part I, but the recent momentum of that technological growth made its expansion inevitable, even entering areas of life where it had little of substance to offer. "This system," says Ellul, "is given to pure growth."[2] Expanding, then, from where it was nearly miraculous in treating diseases to places where it had little to offer, biomedicine—now biohealth—needed to develop characteristics and techniques to give it legitimacy, protect its hegemony, and present its influence as authoritative. Or perhaps it brought these characteristics with it, and they serve it well.

In Part II we will look at the following characteristics of biohealth:

- Biohealth is a *system*. Systems thinking has given us over the last

---

1. Ellul, *Technological Society*, xxv; Stivers. *Technology as Magic*, 17.
2. Ellul, *Technological System*, 117.

generation a vocabulary to think about complex phenomena in our societies. As in any system, no aspect of biohealth can be analyzed or modified alone; all inter-relate. Practitioners of biohealth embrace systems thinking. Biohealth as a system is the subject of chapter 5.

- Biohealth employs the concept of *risk*. One characteristic of the modern world is a recognition of the reality of risk, both risk as danger and risk as opportunity. Biohealth employs risk in both senses, and is the subject chapter 6.

- Biohealth treats *health as a commodity*, just as it treats all of its other products and services as commodities. This is not only in line with the current world market economy, it is also required by it. Chapter 7 looks at health as a commodity.

- Biohealth places *responsibility* for both good and ill health *on the individual*, not on society. Both the individual and society, of course, are important. But as with all of these characteristics, the problem is less in what biohealth emphasizes than in what it ignores. We will explore the role of individual and social responsibility for health in chapter 8.

- Biohealth employs *bioethics* to justify its emphases. Bioethics, while sometimes taking an "outside view" and sometimes criticizing biomedicine, is now very much part of the biohealth system. We will look at how this functions in chapter 9.

- Finally, biohealth *redefines life*. Over the last several centuries we have been both refining and narrowing our definition of life. Throughout most of history we considered nature itself to be alive. Gradually we realized that only certain parts of it were actually "alive"—plants and animals. We then focused on what in those organisms was the life principle, and called it "protoplasm." Now we call that principle "genes." Chapter 10 will look at how biohealth continues this process in redefining life.

Throughout this section, as in the previous chapter, I will be using illustrations from my own medical life—not as key events in the period, but simply as typical examples any one of us could have experienced. If being trained before 1980 offers any advantage, it may be the hidden memory that biohealth is not the only health.

5

Systems

I N EARLY 2008 I visited a prominent eastern US university with a newly redesigned Family Medicine program, intended to "prepare Family Doctors for the future." On a large poster in their department office was a diagram depicting the "patient-centered" model of care. In the center of the diagram was a circle representing the patient; surrounding this central patient were many other circles, each representing one of the services that was available to the patient: nutrition counseling, social services, visiting nurses, physical therapy, psychological counseling, laboratory, imaging, and so on. Among these outer circles, of course, were the Family Doctor as well as the other consultant doctors who may be involved in the patient's care. Implied spokes led from the "hub" patient to each circle on the rim. All circles, including the patient, were the same size.

The diagram, even in its simplicity, spoke volumes. In an older understanding of illness treatment, there would have been two circles, patient and doctor, connected by a line. Smaller "ancillary" circles would have surrounded the doctor, who would call in those as necessary to help the patient. Older still would simply be two circles, doctor and patient. All of these pictures represent models of systems; the newer patient-centered model is an example of a system becoming more complex. In biohealth, we are intentional about seeing ourselves as working in systems. The promotional literature of the program spoke of "teamwork," "operational management," and "strategy implementation," with an optional fourth-year fellowship preparing "leaders" to "organize and administer complex delivery systems."

Later that day I saw the system in action. I went with a faculty member to a small outlying clinic in a poor neighborhood. The faculty member was a native Spanish speaker originally from South America; her first patient was an undocumented alien from Central America. As we entered the examination room we found him sitting up on the examination couch on its paper sheet, looking exposed and scared. He came because he felt weak and thought he was anemic. The doctor's kind and efficient interview uncovered the essence of his story: he was unable to get a job and was having financial problems; his one-year-old child was awakening frequently at night wanting to feed, disrupting his own sleep. On questioning, he admitted that his wife felt he was drinking too much alcohol. A brief exam showed that he was neither pale nor had any other signs of anemia.

For a doctor functioning in a pure biomedical model, the task now would be straightforward: the doctor would need to confirm that anemia was not present, and "reassure" the patient. That, however, would not be very helpful to the weak patient. According to the biopsychosocial model of *diagnosis*, the clinician, aware that weakness could have psychological and social as well as biological causes, would engage the patient in a conversation to identify all the possible causes. The patient-centered model of *treatment* would then go further, suggesting that the patient must be involved in the next step: what to do about the weakness, especially if the problems causing it were social and psychological. That is, patients must be active participants in their own healthcare—in the "center" of it, in fact.

What I saw, however, was an interpretation of patient-centered care I was not expecting, but one that fit the diagram perfectly. The doctor ordered a minimal number of laboratory tests to confirm that anemia was not the problem, and then began discussing with the patient some of the problems he had mentioned. She asked a few more questions about the baby waking up during the night, and suggested that he and his wife did not need to be feeding him every night; she engaged in "supportive counseling" around one of the issues he had identified. Then she asked more about his alcohol drinking and suggested he consider substance-abuse counseling. She found the name and contact information of the nearest counseling center, and as he was leaving gave him the information on how to contact the center.

This patient, as in the diagram, was in the center of an array of services, an entire system of help focused on the patient in the middle—just as he sat perched on the examination couch in the middle of the room. The doctor tried to make available to him all the helping services she could summon, and he remained in the center—but only as a passive recipient. She *had to* offer him what was available, the possibility of alcohol rehabilitation—but it was for a problem *she* had identified, not one he had. In addition, his main problem, not having a job and being in financial trouble, was not dealt with because there was no help in the system of services surrounding him to solve this thorny problem. Yet he was part of the system in the same way the doctor was—each had their place, but neither was a truly independent actor in this system; neither was really free.

Possibly the most basic or overarching characteristic of biohealth is its self-identification as a system. Today that does not seem surprising, or even worth mentioning: *everything* is a system—just as every organization has problems, every person breathes air, and all fish are wet. How does recognizing biohealth as a system help us understand it?

A system is a collection of parts—people, objects, processes—that function together interdependently. None of these parts can be altered or removed without affecting the overall activity of the system. A car is a system; it doesn't run if you remove the carburetor. A factory is a system; it's activity grinds to a halt if there is no one to buy its products. The earth is an ecological system; the polar ice caps begin to melt when greenhouse gasses increase the atmospheric temperature. Though systems and these sorts of observations about them are not at all new, academic reflection on them is. Only since World War II have scholars named and reflected on "general systems theory." Environmental science, the classic "systems" field of study, did not exist as a major area of study when I was I college in the 1960s. It's as though we suddenly discovered that fish were wet.

We have already seen that healthcare—already a very large complex system during the medicalization period—began seeing itself as a system around 1980. Or more accurately, it began seeing the *service it offered* as a system, the biopsychosocial model. Until then, and still today in many places in the world, neither sick people nor their doctors viewed a trip to the clinic as a part of a system. If anyone had bothered to diagram it, it would have been simply the two circles we mentioned above, and the diagram would have offered nothing to the healing relationship.

As there is now more that biomedicine has to offer, however, the relationships between the parts become complex, and we want to understand those connections. We draw diagrams and flow charts to suggest models for these systems; we want to make sure that we have considered every part of the system. Contemporary analytic language mirrors this desire to be complete: we say we want to "capture" each of the relevant aspects. But our language also betrays us: to capture something is to make it captive. In describing or designing a system, we not only want to include every part, we also want to make each part captive, to control it. So in the diagram of circles around the patient hub (which is a biopsychosocial model of *treatment*, not just diagnosis), the patient is in the center, captured by the caring system. Our patient did not think alcohol was his major problem; to him, weakness was, and on exploring further, financial difficulties. But the system offered counseling for alcohol abuse because it had determined this was a treatable problem; stress caused by lack of employment in an undocumented alien was not.

At the dawn of biohealth, in 1984, William Ray Arney and Bernard Bergen saw all this developing, and described it in *Medicine and the Management of Living: Taming the Last Great Beast*.[1] To them, "the last great beast is no longer death, but life," and the job of the system of biomedicine, or what I've called biohealth, is to manage life. "The symbol," they say, "of this new perspective is the 'chronic patient'" whose problems we "manage" rather than cure.

We can see this more clearly when we compare the management of a chronic disease with the treatment of an acute one. There is little need for systems thinking in treating pneumonia with penicillin, or amputating a gangrenous leg. Or more accurately, systems thinking is not necessary to help us *decide* to prescribe the penicillin or amputate the leg, nor for the patient to benefit from them. Producing antibiotics may involve very complex systems, but *using* them rarely does. Likewise carrying out a safe effective surgical operation requires a very smoothly functioning system, but the patient is peripheral to the functioning of that system, and "performs" best when completely unconscious.

Caring for people with chronic conditions, however, is very different. Insulin does not cure diabetes; our Central American patient was

1. Arney and Bergen, *Medicine and the Management of Living*, 97, 105.

not cured of his weakness by being counseled about child-rearing tech-niques and being offered alcohol rehabilitation. The best we can offer him is to help "manage" the stress causing his weakness, as we help diabetics "manage" their blood sugars. But our patients are not anesthetized, and we cannot fix their problems the way surgeons do. They must participate in their own management—a hallmark of the patient centered model that we knew about on some level long before we articulated it. It was perhaps inevitable that we would come to include patients in the *system* of their own management; that we would capture them.

So far, we have only described the inevitable consequences of of-fering patients treatments that do not cure them. They must inject their own insulin or confront their own financial or alcohol problems—or remain ill. However, biohealth does not stop there. The contention of Arney and Bergen is that the system of biohealth seeks to manage (or tame) not only disease and death, but also life itself—the life not only of diseased people, but of *all* people. This is the point at which the *service* of medicine becomes a *system*; where biomedicine becomes biohealth.

Part I summarized some of the developments that led to this change. The earliest we considered was the International Classification of Diseases, an effective, but as we saw limited, tool for gathering large amounts of statistical data on patients. Based on this sort of intense scrutiny of both sick and well people, biomedicine has decided what is normal in people: which characteristics and behaviors and variations and responses are "within normal limits." Biohealth then uses this in-formation to map out an "ideal life course" for each person, an "optimal trajectory" for every patient. But not just for people with chronic dis-eases; now *everyone*, sick or well, has been captured by the health care system; *everyone* is offered a "life course trajectory" suited to their age, sex, and race.[2]

It begins early. Margaret Sanger and Marie Stopes felt that an ideal life trajectory for poor women was to *not* begin—that is, to have fewer children. When women did get pregnant, Joseph DeLee described an ideal life course that had them deliver in a hospital under anesthesia. Biohealth still supports fertility control and a medicalized birth, but more subtly: we make these services available today, adding plenty of scientific proof bolstering our claim that birth control and hospital

2. Arney and Bergen, *Medicine and the Management of Living*, 87, 100, 149.

births are obvious choices because they are simply common sense. They are part of the optimal life trajectory, the system.

Ensuring that people (*all* people) stay on their ideal life trajectory involves what David Armstrong calls Surveillance Medicine, as we saw in chapter 3. Traditionally, before biomedicine saw the services it offered as a system, its offerings were intended for those who defined themselves as ill. It had nothing to offer healthy people. But as biomedicine found, through the intense observation of large groups of people over time, diseases could be identified in their very earliest forms, before patients knew they were ill. Medicine gradually adopted methods of ongoing scrutiny—surveillance—to find the people who were slipping off of their ideal life trajectory, or who had "risk factors" that made them susceptible to slipping off. One of the earliest forms of surveillance was child welfare clinics, employing growth charts that pictorially displayed each child's actual optimal growth trajectory, making graphically clear those children whose growth was not keeping up.[3]

These examples—Sanger, Stopes, DeLee, and child welfare clinics—all are from the early twentieth century, showing that the roots of biohealth reach far back. But they demonstrate only primitive forms of biohealth. Perhaps the reason that these early forms of biohealth emphasized pregnancy and childhood is that these are times of visible development, and therefore times when things could go wrong, and be redirected. Once the person is an adult, it is more difficult to make changes that influence health, and the interventions are likely to be less effective.

However as we have seen, the mid twentieth century brought vaccines and the Pap test; and later in the century more extensive screening. This period of biohealth has proven, through large "high-powered" studies, that surveillance is effective even for adults. Controlling blood pressure and cholesterol in large populations of adults results in real differences in how many people develop heart disease; finding and treating early forms of some cancers in adults reduces the number of people who die from that cancer.

Now the impact of surveillance of adults is less than, say, making C-sections available for obstructed labor, or vaccinating all children for diphtheria or measles. Less, but not absent; it is fine-tuning, compared with the earlier coarse-tuning. Since its value could be proven, surveil-

3. Armstrong, "Rise of Surveillance Medicine," 396–97.

lance became more and more important to ensure that the *system* of biohealth included everyone. Consequently centrally controlled national health systems are more efficient in promoting biohealth than free enterprise systems such as the American one. We will examine risk and surveillance more closely in the next chapter.

This, then, is what systems thinking *does*: it tries to bring all aspects of an endeavor—all the people, machines, processes, and information— together; it tries to capture *everything*. And because there is so much to capture, it engages the service of computers to keep track of all these aspects. Now when the system is a machine, such as a modern passenger jet, the computer does an excellent job of coordinating the information, even to the point of flying the jet with very little input from the pilot. A joke recorded by Arney in another study makes the point well: "Planes in the future will be flown by one pilot and one dog. The pilot will be there to feed the dog and the dog will be there to bite the pilot if he even thinks about touching the controls."[4]

But when the system is made up of people—in fact exists to serve people, as biohealth does—the coordinating role of the computer becomes more ambiguous. This is partly, as we saw in chapter 2, because with computers it is "all but impossible to enter certain kinds of data," and "all but impossible *not* to record other kinds of data."[5] However, as Yves Filion points out, problems with systems thinking go beyond computer management of data. The goal of systems thinking is to be explicit about the connections between the parts, but "certain interconnections within the system take precedence over others because they contribute more directly to the simple result that the system is designed to achieve"—usually related to performance and efficiency. And since "the systems perspective hails from a purely technical, as opposed to cultural, order," human elements can be simply ignored.[6]

Filion is admittedly analyzing business and engineering systems, but his critique raises an ominous question about a system designed to serve humans, as biohealth claims. Can a modern technological system offer and preserve *shalom* health? The computer facilitates the flow of information within biohealth, but "because information can only express the quantitative aspects of what is knowable, it filters out a great many

---

4. Arney, *Experts in the Age of Systems*, 45.

5. Clarke et al., "Biomedicalization," 174.

6. Filion, "Moral Impotence of Contemporary Experts," 345–46.

aspects of human life and the biosphere."[7] But biohealth *focuses* on human life; does this critique apply to biohealth?

Look at the optimal life trajectory and the "management of living" which biohealth offers everyone. Biohealth decides on these trajectories, as we have seen, based on studies that analyze data about large groups of people; it also makes recommendations based on criteria it inherits from systems thinking, criteria related to efficiency, productivity, and maximal use of time and money that the "purely technical" systems approach espouses. Biohealth can thus measure how much longer a man lives after taking its advice (a screening test, for example), but will find it far more difficult to measure how happy that man is during his statistically significantly longer life. Biohealth can prove that a woman who delivers her baby in a hospital will have a higher chance of going home with a live infant, but it has more difficulty proving that a woman who delivers at twenty-four weeks and goes home with a live but damaged baby has made the right choice.

In other words, as biohealth becomes more and more a *technological* system, it comes less and less to resemble a *natural* system such as the ocean, the human body, or a hunter-gatherer tribe. In fact, the problem with biohealth is not that it is a system, but that it is a *technological* system. It is worth looking in some more detail at this distinction to help us understand why this difference is important. As we previously mentioned, Jacques Ellul provided a foundation for understanding modern technology as a system throughout his writings, especially in *The Technological System*[8] and his earlier *The Technological Society.*[9]

Two points are crucial in understanding biohealth as a system. First is what Ellul, and many following him, have meant by technology. The common understanding is that technology refers to tools and machines—and certainly these are included. However, the French word *la technique* (which was in the title of *The Technological Society* in French) actually points to a broader understanding of "technology," the usual English translation of *la technique*. In fact, the English word technique may be closer to what Ellul was talking about. In a "Note to the Reader" written a decade after the original French edition of *The Technological Society* was published, Ellul tried to clarify: "In our technological soci-

7. Ibid.

8. Ellul, *Technological System*.

9. Ellul, *Technological Society*.

ety," he wrote, "*technique* is the *totality of methods rationally arrived at . . . in every* field of human activity."[10] That is, all methods and techniques designed by people ("rationally arrived at") for accomplishing any task are, for Ellul, technology.

In an attempt to make this clear, Ellul separates mechanical techniques from human techniques; his disciple Richard Stivers analyzes several of these human techniques in detail. Stivers calls them "nonmaterial technologies for the control of humans"—or "information technologies," and includes among them "therapy, sales, advertising, mass media programs . . . and administrative techniques like systems analysis and strategic planning."[11] Many of these of course use the technology of machines, but it is important to consider them as technologies in their own right. For example, no machines at all are necessary for psychotherapy, or advertising, or management; but all of these endeavors follow very clear methods, and all seek efficiency.

Efficiency is for Ellul a pivotal characteristic of technology. The full phrase from the "Note to the Reader" mentioned above was "*technique* is the *totality of methods rationally arrived at and having absolute efficiency* (for a given stage of development) in *every* field of human activity.*" When we realize that all methods that people develop to accomplish tasks efficiently can be considered "technology," it is clear that biohealth is right at the center of our technological society.

While efficiency is the defining characteristic of technological systems, it is not the only characteristic Ellul describes. Looking at these other qualities of technology[12] is the second point we can learn from Ellul, and provides a nice concluding summary of biohealth as a system.

Technological systems are automatic and self-augmenting: they go by themselves and they grow by themselves. This is "the technological imperative"—what can be done must be done, and doing it leads to something else. In the process, the new replaces the old, even if the old was perfectly good. We see this all the time in the pharmaceutical industry: newer (more expensive) drugs constantly are replacing other treatments or older drugs, often with minimal or no benefit compared with existing treatments. Many perfectly functional generic blood pressure drugs and antibiotics have been upstaged by newer brand-name devel-

---

10. Ellul, *Technological Society,* xxv; emphasis in the original.

11. Stivers, *Technology as Magic,* 43.

12. Ellul, *Technological Society,* 79–147; Ellul *Technological System,* 125–255.

opments. Metformin is not as good as exercise in preventing diabetes, but it does have some effect;[13] it therefore becomes one of our choices. SSRI antidepressant drugs are no better than exercise in treating depression in older patients[14]—but the standard treatment remains medication, and the option of using exercise for depression is almost unknown to the public.

Technologically-produced new commodities (see chapter 7) always displace existing ways of understanding a problem, and trump existing treatments. The same is true with surgery, as we saw with cosmetic surgery. As the ability to change a person's appearance becomes for some people an imperative, the demand rises—and plastic surgery morphs from being predominantly reconstructive to over half cosmetic.

Another set of characteristics of technological systems is their "totalization," their all-inclusiveness. In fact, says Ellul, there is really just one total technological system, and all subsystems (such as biohealth) are part of it. This super-system embraces all methods and techniques of all human endeavors (sports, medicine, art, religion, agriculture, education, manufacturing, and so forth) everywhere. We saw in chapter 2 how biohealth embraces complementary and alternative medicine; likewise the technological system driven by performance and efficiency embraces biohealth. And although world-wide universality of biohealth (as part of the technological system) is not complete, we will consider in chapter 12 how widespread it has become.

Finally, Ellul emphasizes that the technological system is autonomous; there is no person or committee or government able to hold it in check. In fact, no one is trying, because the benefits, or at least the power, of the technological system are so pervasive. Few would want to halt research for new "life-saving" drugs or surgical procedures. But even when questions are raised about the need for certain research and whether or not it really will lead to "life-saving" procedures, there is no stopping the process: the momentum is too great. Yet this momentum itself points to a unique characteristic of the technological system: it's lack of feedback. All systems except the technological system have feedback loops that keep the system in homeostasis, that are self-correcting. However, the technological system has none: it only grows.

13. Knowler et al., "Reduction in the incidence of type 2 diabetes," 393–403.
14. Blumenthal et al., "Effects of Exercise Training," 2349–56.

Unchecked growth: in healthcare, our biggest concern is growing costs; we are far less concerned about the growth of healthcare itself. In fact, in the US we constantly talk of ways to *expand* coverage while keeping costs down. But unchecked growth is never benign. The essence of one kind of science fiction horror movie is an animal or insect that keeps growing. In biology, we call an unchecked growth cancer.

6

Risk

OVER TWO DECADES AGO Ulrich Beck declared that we live in a "risk society."[1] It's not so much that risk is unique to the modern world, because it isn't. The difference from past ages is that we now think a lot more about risk—and even more importantly, we now very carefully measure it. Measuring and trying to modify risk is a central tenet of biohealth.

But what is risk? The common understanding is that risk has something to do with danger, and on Beck's first page he links risk to the "hazards and potential threats" that have arisen because of the "modernization process." Fair enough: as technology's power increases, its dangers correspondingly increase, as Three Mile Island and Chernobyl have shown us.

However, Anthony Giddens says, "Risk isn't the same as hazard or danger. Risk refers to hazards that are actively assessed in relation to future possibilities."[2] By this definition, the danger of hunting in a traditional society is not risk. It is simply danger, the danger that the wild animal will hurt or kill the hunter, while success in killing the animal only feeds the family and preserves the status quo. The whole endeavor does not open "future possibilities." On the other hand, when Columbus set out across the Atlantic in search of the gold of the Indies, he took a risk: failing might mean death, but succeeding in finding that gold would make him famous and rich.

1. Beck, *Risk Society.*
2. Giddens, *Runaway World,* 22.

Both of these aspects, the danger part and the future possibility part, are deeply woven into how biohealth uses risk, and are best illustrated by a story:

In 1999, after working in East Africa for a decade, my wife Jan and I decided to get tested for AIDS. As doctors who had operated on many patients who might have had AIDS (but didn't know because they hadn't been tested), and knowing we had been stuck occasionally by needles during these surgeries, we realized that there was a small chance, a risk, that one of us had been infected by the HIV virus. We also reasoned that knowing our HIV status had value with respect to "future possibilities": a positive test would imply testing our CD4 counts, eventually taking ARV drugs, and practicing safe sex.

The testing process itself, however, was far riskier than we had imagined. We used the ELISA test to screen ourselves, the same test we used on patients in our Kenyan hospital at the time. Mine came back negative, Jan's positive. We then had her blood tested with the Western Blot test, the gold standard; the result was "indeterminate." The following month was harrowing as we left for an already planned trip to the US to enter our daughter into college. During the trip, Jan had a full set of blood tests including a CD4 count, a repeat Western Blot, and a viral load: all came back negative, with the CD count normal. Jan's positive AIDS test had been a "false positive."

Though we were not infected by AIDS, we had been infected by risk; biohealth had followed us to East Africa. We were aware of the small risk that we could have been infected with HIV without knowing it, and biohealth prescribed for us a way to "control" that risk, a way to open "future possibilities" if one of our tests was positive. But that means of control brought its own risk: needless profound anxiety.

Or was it really needless? We took a risk by taking the test, and a risk by definition implies not knowing the outcome ahead of time. If I smoke cigarettes I risk getting lung cancer—but I might not get it. If I invest money in a new company I risk losing it all—or making a lot more money. If I submit to a screening test, I risk getting an anxiety-producing false positive, or temporary relief with a negative test—temporary because I'll likely feel the need to be tested again next year. But I also might find an early form of a disease I can control before it damages me. In biohealth we confront the uncertainty of a health risk with the uncertainty of a screening test. We fight fire with fire, we use chewing gum to scrape the chewing gum off our shirt. How did this come about?

In previous regimes of biomedicine, certainly before World Wall II but in a large part before 1980 as well, *risk* was not part of our thinking. We certainly knew about hazards and dangers to health; we could observe the cause of behaviors or exposures and the resulting effect of illness. We knew about sexually transmitted disease, we knew that tuberculosis could be caught from someone who had tuberculosis. We discovered more recently that cigarette smoking was hazardous to health; we have know for millennia that war was hazardous to health. But we did not consider any of these as *risks* in the sense of future possibilities (except maybe the hazards of war), and our *calculations* of these dangers were minimal.

Imagine, for a moment, that AIDS first appeared and was described clinically fifty years earlier, in 1931. We might have noticed then, as we did in 1981, that it was a "3H" disease, common in homosexual men, Haitians, and heroin users (blood transfusions were not yet used for the fourth H, hemophiliacs). We would not have known that it was an infectious disease, and would not have been able to prove or test for it by 1933, as we could in 1983. Had my wife and I been alive then, doing surgery on homosexuals, heroin users, or Haitians in the mid 1930s, we would not have known that this surgery carried any additional risk to us. And even if we did wonder, there would have been no way to evaluate our "future possibilities." We would not have seen our activity as risky, and we would not have exposed ourselves to the risk of a false positive test because there would not have been any tests.

What has made the difference in the regime of biohealth is not the character of the disease, but our knowledge about it. But not just our advanced and detailed knowledge; what is different today is the *way* we think. Before biohealth, we broadly understood the connections between cause and effect; now we are fine-tuning those connections. Before biohealth, we thought about those connections qualitatively; now we measure them. Before biohealth, we tried to at least control what we could observe in the present; now we try to control what we cannot see because it has not yet happened. Before biohealth, we confronted danger; now we manage risk.

Risk thinking, like systems thinking, changes how we approach medicine and health. Current epidemiologic studies have shown that the risk of becoming HIV positive after being stuck by a needle from an HIV + patient is about 1 in 300—likely less risky than getting hepatitis in the same way from a hepatitis patient.[3] Had we known this in 1939, we would likely have felt the risk was so low that it wasn't worth considering. Even if treatment was available in 1939, we would probably have chosen to wait to see if we became ill before beginning treatment. But in 1999, risk thinking, and a sense of responsibility (see chapter 8), pushed us to *do something*—not based on feeling ill, but based on the *risk* of falling ill.

This story of our confronting a risk with a screening test illuminates three important facets of risk when it is used in biohealth: it involves probability calculations, it produces anxiety, and it calls for surveillance. We will look at each one in detail.

There is nothing new about the branch of mathematics called probability. Probability calculations were necessary to determine insurance premiums over two hundred years ago. This "trading and off-loading of risk" is an essential feature of our economy; "capitalism is actually unthinkable and unworkable without it."[4] In fact, when applied to large groups, probability calculations are an excellent way to confront the uncertainty of the future. I don't know when I sell Mr. Smith fire insurance if his house will burn down next week—but I can predict that if I sell one hundred fire insurance policies at a certain premium, I can likely pay for the one house that will burn, and still have some left over as profit. I of course don't know, and don't care, if the house that burns will be Mr. Smith's.

The same is true with gambling: from a well-shuffled deck, if I choose a card randomly I have a 25 percent chance of drawing a heart. That is a one in four chance, meaning that if I draw four times, I will probably get one heart. But I may on those first four draws end up with a club, a diamond, and two spades. The more times I draw, the closer to 25 percent will be my collection of hearts. My chance of drawing a red card on the first draw is 50 percent; my chance of *not* drawing a spade is 75 percent. I have definite ways of calculating my *risk* of getting what I want or don't want on the first draw—but not of *determining* what I will get. The more times I draw, the more helpful my probability calculations will be.

3. Ridzon et al., "Simultaneous Transmission of Human Immunodeficiency Virus," 919–22.

4. Giddens, *Runaway World*, 25.

We use exactly the same sort of reasoning in evaluating and calculating risks to our health; we speak of relative risk, relative risk reduction, absolute risk reduction, and odds ratios. All of these calculations are very accurate ways to describe what will happen to a population of people exposed to, say, a radiation leak from a nearby nuclear plant, or for predicting how many women over seventy-five will have a hip fracture in the next year, with different predictions for those who have taken calcium and vitamin D over the last ten years, and those who haven't. However, if I am a seventy-six year old woman who has not been taking calcium and vitamin D, these calculations cannot tell me for sure that I will have a hip fracture in the coming year. They only tell me my *risk*—a calculated number—of fracturing my hip. But I have only one draw from the deck, and as we saw, the risk calculations on that first draw are not very helpful.

Return for a minute to our HIV tests. Had we carefully studied our situation before getting tested, we would have determined that a screening test for us would have a low "predictive value": First, the test itself may have been designed to be so sensitive in picking up HIV that it sometimes even turned positive when there was no HIV. But equally important, the prevalence of the disease in a population of people like us was very low to begin with, meaning a screening test would be less valuable. Or, in statistical language, we were not *assured* of a false positive test, we simply faced a higher *risk* of our tests being false positive. More chewing gum to remove chewing gum from our shirt.

The fundamental question here about probability statistics is how useful they are to a single patient. Probability is indispensable in our economy, in the insurance industry, and in gambling. Likewise in public health, probability statistics are extremely important, and for a clinician, probability statistics are one of several pieces of information I can use in diagnosing and treating patients. But for an individual patient, probability statistics have much more limited use. In fact, they can cause more harm than good, as we will now consider.

The second problem with risk thinking is the anxiety it can produce. Social scientists have repeatedly recognized and analyzed this since the beginning of contemporary risk thinking. In *Risk Society*, Ulrich Beck said, "The movement set in motion by the risk society . . . is expressed in the statement: *I am afraid!*"[5] Around the same time, a British study asked

5. Beck, *Risk Society*, 49.

"Can health screening damage your health?" and concluded that there was "a significant increase in psychological distress in healthy adults who have been screened for coronary heart disease risk factors."[6] Fifteen years later Robert Crawford extensively analyzed this anxiety in "Risk ritual and the management of control and anxiety in medical culture."[7]

Theoretically, identifying risks early and dealing with them before they become aggressive diseases should make us healthier and happier. So why does risk thinking produce anxiety? There are at least two reasons. The first we have seen: if a test result of a risk factor is not definitive, we can get anxious wondering what the result means, and whether the next one will be positive. Positive tests give us anxiety about the diseases they have identified; we cannot retrospectively erase that anxiety when those tests were *false* positives. It is still real anxiety, but because there is no real object of that anxiety, it is needless anxiety.

The second reason comes closer to the heart of biohealth. In the regime of biohealth, health increasingly becomes what biomedicine can offer us. As biomedicine uncovers more and more of the molecular and genetic bases for disease, and especially as it fine-tunes these discoveries, we are confronted with huge amounts of information about the earliest forms of disease—or pre-disease, or just the statistical risk factors for disease. As the amount of information increases, our threshold for concern falls: should we act on this new study? create a screening program based on this discovery? recommend or take medication or change our behavior to reduce the newly identified risk factor?

The presence of all of this information is itself anxiety-producing: how can we process all of this? As providers, we have a somewhat easier job: we increasingly use electronic records, and divide our tasks so that some of us focus more on actual and advanced disease (hospitalists and specialists), and others on early or potential disease (primary care specialists). But patients and potential patients cannot divide themselves up this way: all of us in the regime of biohealth are now expected to pursue health as well as financial security and happiness. We must now not only confront the financial and security risks people have always faced, but we must also face the health risks that biohealth increasingly makes us aware of. It is no surprise that we become more anxious.

6. Stoate, "Can Health Screening Damage your Health?" 193–95.
7. Crawford, "Risk Ritual," 505–28.

What is surprising, however, is this: though we are more aware of health risks than in previous eras, there are probably no more actual risks to health than there have ever been. In fact, in rich industrialized countries at least, there continue to be measurable improvements in the health status of the populations—but those improvements "have not been accompanied by improvements in the subjective feeling of healthiness and physical well-being." On the contrary, "people now report higher rates of disability, symptoms, and general dissatisfaction with their health."[8] One of the reasons for this paradox is the risk thinking we have been discussing.

Before discussing how to respond to this anxiety, it is worth considering how biomedicine usually confronts this sort of problem. We have just suggested that "risk society"—a society in which risk thinking affects everything we do—results in increased overall anxiety, or at least the lack of "improvements in the subjective feeling of healthiness." But is this true? Is there proof?

Biomedicine approaches this question the way it approaches every other question: it selects a specific disease for which we have identified risk factors—diabetes for example—and then divides potential diabetics into two groups, those who are subjected to risk thinking (are screened or given advice), and those who aren't. It then tests both groups for anxiety. If there is no difference in the anxiety of the two groups, the study concludes that the particular form of risk thinking used for the particular disease does not increase anxiety.[9]

Now look more closely at the way biomedicine asks the question: with a microscope. It narrows its focus onto a tiny measurable example of the larger question. When it joins together many of these studies in a meta-analysis, it purports to provide a satellite view. But it is not a satellite view; it is a multi-microscopic view. It assumes that the whole is only the sum of the parts.

These sorts of studies have in fact provided mixed results: some confirm that attention to risk increases anxiety; some don't. On balance, however, writers for the *British Medical Journal*, using studies like these, concluded that "screening could seriously damage your health."[10] This

8. Barsky, "Paradox of Health," 414–18.

9. Pierce et al., "More Good than Harm," 867–71.

10. Stewart-Brown and Farmer, "Screening Could Seriously Damage your Health," 533.

was an editorial, not a meta-analysis; it was an attempt at a satellite view. It was *opinion*. Other satellite views come from artists, philosophers, and theologians—but their methods and assumptions are so different from scientists that combining the conclusions of both becomes very difficult.

In between the two approaches are the social scientists. They are scientists with their own rigorous methods, but with this difference: their unit of focus is society, not atoms or cells or organs or individual people. Biomedicine may debate whether or not a specific screening test increases anxiety, but social scientists ask questions of the nature of society itself. Consequently, Robert Crawford could *begin* his analysis of anxiety in the medical culture of risk with this statement, "My contention is that a distinctive feature of contemporary medical culture is *an escalating spiral of control and anxiety*."[11] He *contends* this at the beginning, and proceeds to argue his case throughout the article.

This is the satellite view of a social *scientist*—but medical practitioners do not comb the social science literature the way they comb the biomedical literature. Hence, the points of departure of social scientists are not always assumed by biomedical practitioners. Doctors and social scientists each have their own language and conventions as well their own methods of research. Scholars may be comfortable traversing both medicine and medical sociology, but few practicing doctors are. Clinicians who see anxious patients wait for the meta-analyses to "prove" why these patients are anxious.

While it may be true, then, that specific screening tests do not always produce anxiety, our age is nevertheless characterized by a restlessness, a "general dissatisfaction" with health. We may not be able to "prove" it, but Crawford's contention, that this anxiety is in some way related to our constant awareness of risks to our health, seems reasonable. How does biohealth respond to this anxiety?

One response might be to remove the "offending agent"—but this is impossible if the offending agent is risk itself. Another is to "treat" the anxiety—comparable to giving aspirin to lower the fever of a patient with bacterial pneumonia. This is compassionate and necessary, but incomplete. The sort of "microscopic" studies mentioned above suggest a third approach: redesign screening interventions so that they are less anxiety-producing. For biohealth this approach has the advantage

11. Crawford, "Risk ritual," 506 (emphasis in the original).

of preserving the benefits of risk thinking by fine-tuning the response, without having to question the underlying assumption of risk.

When taken on a larger scale, this perfecting of the screening tools becomes the "surveillance medicine" we mentioned in the last chapter. Armstrong says that Surveillance Medicine established "that everyone was normal yet no-one was truly healthy," a hallmark of biohealth. Extensive studies of large groups of people have identified a wide range of "normality," but all of those "normal" people are at risk of becoming ill, and therefore abnormal. Biohealth has much to offer those on the way to becoming ill, but it must first identify them. In fact, "Surveillance Medicine [and therefore biohealth] requires the dissolution of the distinct clinical categories of healthy and ill as it attempts to bring everyone within its network of visibility. . . . in Surveillance Medicine illness becomes a point of perpetual becoming."[12]

Although Armstrong demonstrates that the roots of Surveillance Medicine date to the early years of the twentieth century, they were only roots then. When I was in medical school in the 1970s, I was still being taught "chief complaint medicine"—that is, the beginning of every encounter between a patient and a clinician was the "chief complaint" of the patient. The first focus was on what was wrong *from the patient's point of view*. We knew about risk and screening programs, but we were not taught to assume that every apparently well person was "perpetually becoming" ill. Most of us trained then have subsequently learned that biohealth expects us to be vigilant in looking for people who do not yet know they are ill; to hunt down "the last well person."[13] Surveillance Medicine (with its connotation of "surveillance camera") was fully operational by 1984, the year George Orwell suggested for the society of "Big Brother Is Watching You."

Let us return to HIV testing for an example. My wife and I decided to get tested because we felt we had a small risk of being infected. Had we been agriculturalists or educators it would not have occurred to us to get tested. However, according to Surveillance Medicine, *everyone* is at risk for getting AIDS; everyone should be tested, especially in Africa. The cornerstone of AIDS prevention in Africa has moved from ABC (Abstinence, Be faithful, use a Condom) to VCT (Voluntary Counseling and Testing). "Know your status" is the rallying cry. Our district hos-

12. Armstrong, "Rise of Surveillance Medicine," 395, 402.

13. Meador, Clifton, "Last Well Person," 440–41.

pital in rural Kenya sported a poster in 2008 of American presidential aspirant Barak Obama and his wife Michelle getting their AIDS tests. Knowing your HIV status has become as important as knowing your birth date.

Unfortunately, knowing your status has upstaged actual prevention. Surveillance has triumphed, selling itself as the first tool of prevention. But prevention is still ABC; knowing your status does not prevent AIDS, avoiding the virus does.[14] VCT is quintessential Surveillance Medicine. The argument, of course, is that those who know they are positive will practice safer sex (thereby reducing HIV spread), and present themselves for regular blood testing in preparation for life-long anti-retroviral drugs (ARVs) when they need them. And those who know they are negative will . . . practice safer sex in an attempt to stay negative. Clearly, then, practicing safer sex does not require knowing your status. VCT may be a tool to collect people and offer them ARVs, and it can be an epidemiological tool for tracking the prevalence of AIDS in a community. But who does this surveillance primarily benefit? We will return to this biohealth approach to AIDS in Africa as a case study in chapter 12.

14. See also Scott and Freeman, "Prevention as a Problem of Modernity," 156.

7

Commodities

I RECENTLY RECEIVED A PROMOTIONAL leaflet[1] for health screening in my junk mail. The leaflet asked "Should you take these life saving tests?" and went on to briefly describe five "painless tests" that were "so important." Three of them were ultrasound tests for atherosclerotic plaques in arteries; those, together with a fourth for atrial fibrillation, comprised the "Stroke, Vascular Disease, & Heart Rhythm Package" which cost $139—not covered by insurance or Medicare "without the presence of symptoms." The company offering the tests found this refusal to pay "unfortunate since *there are often no symptoms for the diseases for which we screen.*" For only ten additional dollars customers could add a fifth ultrasound test for osteoporosis, a condition that is "painless and silent in its early stages." The motto of the company, written under its name, was "The Power of Prevention."

At first glance, the services offered seem useful in our "risk society"—or at least benign. Stroke and other vascular diseases are major killers in the US, and the tests being offered are painless, free of radiation exposure, give immediate answers, and involve little time and no embarrassment. And for middle class or professional people, the cost may be no more than a weekend dinner with a few friends at a fancy restaurant. That may be the way the sensible, informed (and financially well-off) people who want to be responsible about their health might see this screening "package."

However, there are flaws woven throughout this form of Surveillance Medicine. Just under the question on the front of the leaflet asking if the

1. Life Line Screening.

88

reader should take these tests is some advice: "Don't hesitate to ask your doctor." If the doctor being consulted is familiar with recommendations of the US Preventive Services Task Force (USPSTF),[2] that doctor would recommend *against* three of the tests offered in the leaflet, and suggest one of them only for men over sixty-five who have smoked (abdominal aortic aneurysm screening), and the other only for women over sixty-five (osteoporosis).

For one of the tests *not* recommended by the USPSTF (peripheral arterial disease), there is the chilling comment in the leaflet that "it is 4–5 times more likely you will die from heart disease if you have peripheral arterial disease." The promoters of screening are clearly using the anxiety generated by this risky situation to scare people into their surveillance package. However, in this case the only thing they have to offer is anxiety, as there is little evidence (according to the USPSTF) that treating this asymptomatic disease improves health outcomes. And of course the screening test could be a false positive, leading to further unnecessary tests and anxiety—and even the possibility of iatrogenic disease from unnecessary interventions.

Finally we return to the motto of the company: "The Power of Prevention." As we saw in chapter 3, screening is only *secondary* prevention; *primary* prevention is keeping a disease from happening in the first place. Yet the leaflet addresses these more fundamental issues of primary prevention only in small print at the end, granting the need for "appropriate modification of stroke risk factors." Five are listed, including "poor diet"; lack of exercise is not listed. Using the motto "The Power of Prevention" on a leaflet about screening reinforces this conflation of ideas characteristic of biohealth: prevention = screening.

We noted this earlier. However, we are now ready to consider why, to see the medically controlled activities of screening in a larger context. Before medicalization, prevention was the *activities* people did (or did not do) to live a healthy life. It was also, in a larger sense, the norms that society enforced, sometimes legally, to engender health: Prohibition is a classic example, as are building codes requiring indoor plumbing. However, people did not rely on things they *bought* in order to remain healthy. They bought things to eat, to wear, to move with, and to have fun—but health was not for sale. Health has never been a commodity.

---

2. US Department of Health and Human Services, USPSTF website.

Until now. The gradual intrusion of commodities and the market into more and more areas of our lives is a characteristic of the time following World War II. Ivan Illich saw how extensive this was becoming, and in 1978 published a small book looking at this commodification.[3] He compared the increasing use of market commodities to satisfy human needs with the experience of people living in subsistence economies. "The multiplication of commodities and dependence on them," he wrote, "have forcibly substituted standardized packages for almost everything people formerly did or made on their own . . . Plastic had replaced pottery, carbonated beverages replaced water, Valium replaced chamomile tea, and records replaced guitars." Pottery and guitars were certainly goods that could be sold; they were commodities. But they could usually be made locally. Plastic containers and phonograph records were only made in factories; they were not part of a subsistence economy.

This was in 1978, at the beginning of the regime of biohealth. Medicalization was already riding on this wave of commodities, as we have seen: drugs for deviant behavior, cosmetic surgery, and of course screening tests. Now using commodities *to treat disease* is not itself a problem; subsistence economies by themselves could not purify penicillin, isolate insulin, or build, equip, and staff modern operating rooms. Diabetics die without insulin; women with ruptured ectopic pregnancies die without surgery. But thirsty people do not die if they lack carbonated beverages; people with large noses do not die if they lack cosmetic surgery. The problem is not commodities, but commodification: the linking of all needs and wants with market-produced commodities to satisfy them.

We begin to see this more clearly by looking again at the company offering ultrasound screening tests. The company, which profits from selling these commodities, does not make clear how few of these tests lead to an improvement in health. It sells what people will buy, and how much it sells depends on how successful it is in convincing people that their desire for health can be satisfied by the tests. The USPSTF, on the other hand, is based not on profit but on evidence, defined as what scientific studies have shown. The company side-steps this evidence, not by lying about it, but by ignoring it. It sells to people what they want to buy—and its advertising helps create those wants. Arnold Relman

---

3. Illich, *Right to Useful Unemployment*, 24, 27. See also Lander, *Defective Medicine*, "The Commodification of Healing," 92–100.

called this marketing of healthcare services a "new medical-industrial complex" in an article published in the prestigious *New England Journal of Medicine*—in 1980.[4]

Commodities in healthcare, then, are not new; what is new since the 1980 watershed is that health itself has now become a commodity. Relman referred mostly to disease care companies (proprietary hospitals, private laboratories, renal dialysis) in his 1980 analysis. But the company that sent me the leaflet was focused on diseases where "there are often no symptoms," diseases that are "painless and silent"; in other words, it was targeting people who were apparently healthy. Being painless and symptom-free could, of course, mean that I have no disease. In fact it usually does. But in our risk society, we are increasingly aware that I *might* have a disease. Consequently, to ensure my health, I purchase screening tests. I have effectively purchased the newest commodity, health.

We purchase health as a commodity in may other ways: health foods, diet jams and soft drinks, vitamin supplements, membership in a gym, home exercise machines, running shoes and sweat suits, self-help books . . . It is a long list of commodities, none of which improve our health more than walking every day, eating fresh fruits and vegetables, and having friends. But are there commodities that we should purchase to maintain our health? What about the screening tests that the USPSTF *does* recommend based on evidence?

The question is well worth engaging, as it helps us to probe deeper into the nature of health itself. Evidence, as we saw above, is what scientific studies tell us. These studies are experiments, often involving two groups of people that are treated differently; the studies are set up to answer specific questions. But evidence of this sort comes with caveats. If there is a difference between the two groups, what caused it? Is the difference big enough to matter? It is widely accepted that during the period of Prohibition, fewer people died from alcoholic cirrhosis. But did banning alcohol cause this reduction? And even if it did, is that the only question that matters? How do we explain that during the same period, the US homicide rate rose?[5]

Similar questions arose much more recently regarding whether or not all menopausal women should take replacement hormones.

4. Relman, "New Medical-Industrial Complex," 963–70.
5. Miron, "Alcohol Prohibition," 16th paragraph.

Menopause is a normal event, the end of the time of fertility which began with an equally normal event, menarche. But menopause can be accompanied by uncomfortable physical symptoms—as can menarche—and it heralds a time of increased risk for some diseases, especially heart disease and osteoporosis. Since that increased risk comes from decreasing estrogen production, researchers proposed (and found evidence for) giving all menopausal women hormone replacement. However, further studies showed that while there were benefits to the bones and heart, there were risks of increased breast cancer for women who took hormones. The advice depended on which question was asked—did estrogen help the heart and bones, or did estrogen increase the incidence of cancer?

We can ask whether or not acting on a screening test or taking a drug reduces mortality, and a well-designed study will tell us. We can also ask whether following a certain diet or activity pattern throughout life can reduce mortality—a study more difficult to perform, but if done well, will also give us evidence. But it is not just that the first study is easier to perform. Evidence for a screening test or drug in the first study implies the availability of that test or drug: commodities. Evidence for a certain food or activity pattern implies societal norms or individual responsibility, which we will examine closely in the next chapter. As our leaflet showed, someone can make money from selling screening tests, as long as the advertising is convincing; no one makes money from promoting individual responsibility or changing society.

Listening to evidence is certainly more sensible than listening to advertising, but this sort of scientific evidence cannot be the final word. While advertising gives an overall picture that may be skewed or even false, evidence gives a very focused microscopic picture that, while "true," may be skewed because it is so focused. Combining microscopic evidence may work for disease care (the multi-microscopic view we considered in the previous chapter), but is less valuable for understanding *health*, which as we saw in the first chapter means wholeness. We can consider all the evidence that science presents us with. But we must pause when "evidence" suggests that we need a commodity in order to remain healthy, for that would suggest that health was not possible before that commodity was available.

Another place where we see the influence of the market and commodities in biohealth is the practice, in the US and New Zealand at least, of direct to consumer advertising of prescription drugs. Advertising is a pivotal element in ensuring that commodities available on the market get sold. As we saw earlier, the US Federal Trade Commission declared at the dawn of biohealth that the AMA's restriction of advertising doctors' services amounted to a restraint of trade (thereby making clear that what doctors offered was a commodity). About the same time adverts began appearing for prescription drugs in US general readership magazines.[6] Fifteen years later the US FDA issued guidelines about direct to consumer advertising of prescription drugs for the broadcast media, resulting in a marked increase in such advertising on US television over the last decade.[7]

Drugs of course *are* commodities, and in the market, commodities need to be advertised. But there are some "unique features of the medical marketplace, not the least of which is the heavy, often total, dependence of the consumer (patient) on the advice and judgment of the physician." Therefore, "some of the economist's usual assumptions about the competitive free market do not apply to medical care. . . . Unlike consumers shopping for most ordinary commodities, patients do not often decide what medical services they need—doctors usually do that for them."[8] Arnold Relman wrote that in 1980, before direct to consumer advertising of prescription drugs began. This was also a time, as we have seen, when the world was turning more and more to the market for solutions to any problem. During the 1990s the US tried, and failed, to use market solutions for rising healthcare costs and falling healthcare coverage. Relman, it seems, was right—but instead of heeding him we have opened the door even wider to market influence.

While direct to consumer advertising of prescription drugs consumes only about 15 percent of the overall the pharmaceutical advertising budget (the rest is focused on health care providers), looking at *which* drugs are promoted this way provides another interesting window into biohealth. Roughly two-thirds of the adverts for prescription drugs promoted directly to the public in magazines are for symptom relief (allergies, erectile dysfunction, pain, etc). Only one-fourth are for drugs for diagnosed disease (diabetes, hypertension, infections), and the rest are

6. Woloshin et al., "Direct-to-consumer advertisements," 1141–46.

7. Donohue et al., "Decade of Direct-to-Consumer Advertising," 673–81; Rosenthal et al., "Promotion of Prescription Drugs to Consumers," 498–505.

8. Relman, "New Medical-Industrial Complex," 966.

for preventive medicines.[9] Looking at overall drug company spending on advertising, including television, prescription drugs promoted follow a similar pattern, with symptom relief drugs (for heartburn, allergies, pain, and mild depression) usually among the top five. However, preventive medicines (for high cholesterol) are also among these top five.[10]

In other words, direct to consumer advertising for prescription drugs—those that consumers cannot buy without a doctor's permission—is focused precisely on drugs we don't *need*. On reflection, that should be no surprise. Though advertising literally means to make known a commodity and to promote it, that promotion is most important in two situations. Obviously where there is a competing commodity for the same purpose, the manufacturer wants the customer to chose its product; these are the drugs for diagnosed diseases that make up one fourth of direct to consumer advertising. But direct to consumer advertising is primarily informing us about commodities that are designed to do something we don't know we need. This is obvious for the new diseases such as social phobia that we considered in the medicalization chapter. But far more common is the promotion of drugs for common symptoms—mild pain, nasal allergies, erectile dysfunction, heartburn, anxiety or mild depression—that are not dangerous, symptoms that usually do not lead to other conditions and which people throughout history have learned to live with. The same is true with drugs for prevention: we don't *need* them to live. They don't keep us from dying, they only reduce our *risk* of getting certain diseases. Advertising is designed to create needs.

We must be clear about what needs are. I don't *need* relief of my stuffy nose in order to live, work, worship, or converse. If I am a man in my sixties I don't *need* to have sex three times a week. Of course when there is a commodity that can open my nose or regularly give me erections, I may want that commodity. Before it was available, I may not have realized that a stuffy nose or decreasing frequency of sex was a problem; I didn't *need* the commodity that "fixed" those "diseases." When I regularly use those commodities, I miss them when they are not available; I may say that I "need" them. I have therefore become more needy be-

9. Woloshin et al., "Direct-to-Consumer Advertisements," 1142–43.

10. Rosenthal et al., "Promotion of rescription Drugs to Consumers," 498–505; Donohue et al., "Decade of Direct-to-Consumer Advertising," 673–81.

cause they are available—and since the essence of poverty is neediness, I have become poorer.[11]

Though biohealth would claim the opposite, it actually increases our sense of poverty. The core of biohealth is this—health that we achieve by applying the findings of the biological sciences, often in the form of commodities. Those technological advances do not, of course, promote *shalom*; they are not meant to. They are only able to modify our biological mechanics: to relieve our symptoms certainly, but also to change the courses of our diseases. We can be grateful for that, but we should not assume that relieving symptoms or removing disease automatically results in health. The problem is not in using commodities to feel better, it is in substituting commodities for health. If I understand health to be something other than the offerings of biomedicine, I don't need those offerings in order to be healthy. But the degree to which I need biomedicine for health—that is, biohealth—is a measure of my own poverty.

We have until now been considering the commodities that biohealth offers: screening tests and drugs as well as vitamin supplements and running shoes. We have suggested that as a result we come to view health itself as a commodity, a thing we can buy in the medical marketplace—and increasingly a thing we must buy. Before concluding our discussion of commodities we need to look at the other side: the commodities that worsen our health. In the chapter on risk we looked briefly at the hazards of modern life, and clearly nuclear power plants and fast automobiles have their health hazards. However, far more dangerous for far more people in industrial nations, and increasingly is developing nations as well, is the food industry.[12] An automobile is not a human need, but food is—and when the technological system transforms food from a marketable commodity (which it has always been) into an item with "value-added" properties that raise the profit to the seller and decrease the quality for the consumer, the results are lethal.

Possibly the clearest example is the world-wide diabetes epidemic. It is well known that unlike type 1 diabetes, type 2 commonly occurs in overweight people who are sedentary. It is frequently accompanied by high blood pressure and high cholesterol. Consequently, health education for both prevention and treatment focuses on increasing exercise and diet change: fewer calories and fats, and more fiber. That

11. Illich, *Right to Useful Unemployment*, 57–64.
12. See Nestle, *Food Politics*.

makes sense, assuming that the reasons for the inactivity and poor diet are known and addressed. Sometimes they are known.[13] Unfortunately, since these reasons are complex and far deeper than an individual's choice, they are usually not addressed. It should be no surprise that this approach of changing diet and exercise has only marginal success.

It is possible to consider the deeper reasons by looking at changes in the US food supply over the twentieth century. The traditional US diet before World War II relied heavily on whole grains as a major source of carbohydrates. After the war, however, consumption of whole grains began falling, meaning both total carbohydrate and total fiber intake fell. In the 1970s, however, the intake of ready-to-eat cereals began increasing, and beginning in 1980 there was a sharp increase in the consumption of corn syrup, often as a sweetener in other processed foods. Both mean that total caloric intake increased. But there was no corresponding increase in fiber intake. Paralleling these changes was a marked increase in the prevalence of obesity, roughly doubling since 1980—and of type 2 diabetes, which has tripled since the 1960s.[14]

It could, of course, be argued that people *choose* to eat Fruit Loops rather than whole wheat porridge, corn syrup-sweetened ice cream rather than yogurt, and Pepsi rather than fruit juice—and that they could as easily choose not to. But that is a disingenuous argument. People did not demand the food industry to refine corn into sweet syrup, or to remove the nutrients and fiber from wheat in making white flour. The food industries did this—and then advertised and sold these products cheaply to people: "In countries such as the US, it is less expensive (and easier) to buy unhealthy foods."[15] In industrialized countries where most people do not eat what they grow themselves, they buy what is readily available and cheap. There are of course valid arguments for processing foods: ease of transport, less spoilage, etc. But these arguments cannot excuse the food industries from making, promoting, and selling foods that contribute to a massive diabetes epidemic.

We *have* excused them, however. We are beginning to find the tobacco industry culpable, but that is easy because nobody *needs* cigarettes. We all need food, though. So we place the responsibility to eat properly on the individual—and encouraging that responsibility has

13 Yamada and Palafox, "On the Biopsychosocial Model," 702–4.

14. Gross et al., "Increased Consumption of Refined Carbohydrates," 774–79.

15. Yach et al., "Epidemiologic and Economic Consequences," 65.

become the focus of "the new public health." We have just introduced the next chapter.

8

Responsibility

A KEY COMPONENT OF BIOHEALTH is "the belief that individuals can control their own health."[1] In this biohealth regime they of course need *commodities* to help them manage their health *risks* in the context of a healthcare *system*. But underneath, biohealth assumes that each individual can—and must—control their own health. It is their responsibility. Today most of us do not doubt this any more than we doubt the existence of systems or the primacy of risk in understanding health. But today's assumptions are recent, characteristic especially of the post-1980 period.

Immediately before then, in the period of medicalization, responsibility for one's own health had not yet taken preeminence; in fact, biomedicine itself claimed that responsibility—and authority. Biomedicine had grown successful because it focused on discrete causes of illness; in the late nineteenth century germs, and later "distinct, well-defined biochemical or physiological abnormalities"—a "doctrine of specific etiology."[2] This approach also served medicalization well: biomedicine always had something to offer to correct those discrete abnormalities, even if they were not the primary reason for a dis-ease.

A doctrine of specific etiology has always been too narrow, too reductionistic to fully understand ill health and address it. We considered this briefly in the section on the biopsychosocial model. Changing biological mechanisms can reduce symptoms, but rarely gets at the underlying causes of disease (which may be in some measure genetic, but likely in a larger measure economic and political). This truth is some-

1. Galvin, "Disturbing Notions of Chronic Illness," 110.
2. Lander, *Defective Medicine*, 79. See also Tesh, *Hidden Arguments*, chs. 3 and 7.

times masked when treating bacterial infections, because using antibiotics can be so satisfying that we can neglect to ask why the person got the infection in the first place. However, the growth of chronic diseases, and the more limited success of biomedicine in curing them ("A long illness mocks the doctor"[3]), has pushed us to ask the larger questions: why can't we cure these diseases? And where did they come from?

Probably the official launching of our current approach was in the Canadian government's 1974 Lalonde Report which named "lifestyle" along with human biology, the environment, and the health care organization as important determinants of health. This marked the shift from traditional public health, which focused mostly on infectious diseases and epidemic control, to "the new public health," which took under its wing chronic diseases as well. The proposed approach in this report was "health promotion"—but certainly in the context of also addressing social and environmental factors.[4]

In 1977, however, another herald of biohealth, Dr. John Knowles, "threw down the gauntlet which sparked this debate [about individuals controlling their own health] in his article 'The responsibility of the individual'. He claimed that the escalating health care bill in the USA was the result of individual behavioural mismanagement."[5] He was not the first to suggest that how we live has something to do with our health, but his language—"sloth, gluttony, alcoholic intemperance, reckless driving, sexual frenzy and smoking"—certainly captured our attention.

By the time he threw down his gauntlet, Dr. Knowles was already a bit of a celebrity, which may partially explain why his comments attracted such attention. In 1962, at age thirty-six, he became director of the prestigious Massachusetts General Hospital in Boston. In 1969 President Nixon selected him to be the assistant secretary for health in HEW, the nation's top health post. He was clearly energetic, bright—and bombastic: he criticized politicians "who say they want to help poor people and then cut back Medicaid"; his advocacy of "comprehensive, prepaid health insurance" grew from his observation that "if the private basis will not do it, then I think the Federal Government has got to do it." None of this sounds very radical today—but Congress had only re-

---

3. Ecclesiasticus 10:10.

4. Galvin, "Disturbing Notions of Chronic Illness," 109. See also Leeder, "New Public Health."

5. Galvin, "Disturbing Notions of Chronic Illness," 110.

cently created Medicare and Medicaid over the opposition of the AMA, which saw "socialized medicine" everywhere except in private practice. The AMA felt Knowles to be too liberal, and a five-month-long fight ensued. It was an early test of Nixon's leadership, a test he fumbled. Nixon withdrew Knowles's name without ever sending it to Congress for ratification.[6]

Instead of a government post, Knowles became president of the Rockefeller Foundation in 1972. It was during his tenure there, three years later, that he spoke at my medical school graduation. I don't remember his speech, but I do remember the effect that his approach eventually had on me. He was not saying anything new; we already knew that emphysema and lung cancer showed up in people who smoked, alcoholic cirrhosis in people who drank alcohol excessively, gonorrhea in those with multiple sexual partners. Medical school had taught us the mechanisms, but Knowles connected the dots and proclaimed as medical and epidemiological facts what we knew as social facts. He also said publicly what many of us felt like saying individually to our patients: "If you hadn't smoked, you wouldn't be in this situation today!"

His message of individual responsibility for health was very attractive, seductive even. And on one level, for some diseases, it was true. However, medical sociologists saw immediately that in identifying the cause of a person's disease with that person's behavior, there would be a side effect of blaming the sick person for his or her own illness. The titles of Robert Crawford's articles at the time summarized this position: "You are dangerous to your health: The ideology and politics of victim blaming" (1977), and "Sickness as sin: A health ideology for the 1970s" (1978).[7] Blaming the victim not only lacks compassion, it also risks ignoring other factors—social, political, cultural, environmental—that may contribute to the disease causation.

However, despite the early appearance of the victim-blaming critique, these sentiments did not catch hold in the medical world, a world just then entering the regime of biohealth. Biohealth concerns the sort of health achieved by the contributions of the *biological* sciences, not the social, political, and environmental sciences. Biohealth grows out of medicalization, not politicization. And biohealth is very much part of

6. Kotlowski, "Knowles Affair," 443–62.

7. Galvin, "Disturbing Notions of Chronic Illness," 110.

the market-driven post-1980 world, a world in which individualism is the reigning ideology.

This claim bears comment. It is difficult to identify the contemporary world as "individualistic" if we have no reference point, no other society to compare to. However, throughout much of history and in large parts of the world today, the individual was not the fundamental basic unit; the ethnic group or community or family was. People made, and in many places still make, decisions not simply based on personal choice or whim, but in the context of other people who know them, within a culture they hold in common. They in fact "become humans . . . through the process of living in society." When fundamental social groupings no longer carry this authority, we are left with individualism, which assumes that "each person is essentially self-interested and motivated solely by a desire to gain pleasure and avoid pain." The "relevant features" of individuals are "selfishness and competitiveness."[8]

Of course this change from communal living to individualism does not occur overnight and is rarely complete; we all still rely on families and friends for emotional support and direction. But our economics and our ethics betray how far we have moved. In economics, the pared-down individual is a competitive selfish person, the foundation of a free-market economy. And in bioethics, one of the foundational principles—some say *the* foundational principle—is autonomy: the individual is the ultimate authority for anything that biomedicine wishes to offer him or her. Likewise that individual bears ultimate responsibility for his or her own health.

The logic is clear, present among both liberals and conservatives: "Unhealthy behavior results from individual choice . . . so the way to change such behavior is to show people the error of their ways and urge them to act differently."[9] *You* ordered the double cheese-burger; you should order a salad next time. You bought the cigarettes—just don't buy them again. If the TV is on, you can turn it off and go for a walk. The response to the excess of unhealthy commodities produced and sold under Reaganomics was ironically articulated succinctly by Nancy Reagan: "Just say no."

Given a commodity culture, "just say no" is an essential part of that culture that is needed to keep it from damaging our health. For example:

8. Tesh, *Hidden Arguments*, 158.
9. Tesh, *Hidden Arguments*, 161–62.

the automobile industry routinely sells cars with speedometers that go up to 100 MPH, reflecting how fast those cars can go. Most roads are not made for cars to go that fast, and laws prohibit that speed because it is not safe. Yet we continue to make cars more powerful than they need to be, just as we continue to make cigarettes and continue to refine corn into syrup and continue to make handguns and market them to the general public. These free-market items reflect our "free" society: we are free to buy whatever we can afford. If using these things excessively proves dangerous to our health, we should just say no to that excess. Responsibility is the antidote to unhealthy commodities.

But why do we make these things in the first place? Jacques Ellul claimed throughout his writings that there is a technological imperative; that in technology, whatever we can do we will do. We don't make faster cars because we need to in order to solve a problem; we make them because we can. Technology must grow—and therefore fits hand in glove with a market economy that must grow. Prohibiting the development and sale of more and more powerful (or refined, or dangerous) commodities would mean putting the brakes on economic growth, which is not an acceptable option in the post-1980 world. Besides, if Ellul is right, it would not work anyway to prohibit the growth of technology: the technological system is self-augmenting, it grows by itself. It begins to become clear why we pile the responsibility for the misuse of dangerous commodities on the victim rather than on the one who makes the commodity: in our world economy, we cannot control the producer, so we try to control the consumer.

But perhaps this frames the issue too starkly by focusing only on commodities. Perhaps we should talk about responsibility in how we act, not just in what we use. Do we overeat and under-exercise *only* because of cheap poor-quality food, cars, televisions, and computer games? Or, turning it around the other way: isn't it our responsibility to do those things that lead to health, both individually—whether swimming or screening—and cooperatively, through "community participation"? *Community* participation (or community control) may seem to be the opposite of *individual* responsibility for health, and in some important ways it is, drawing as it does from the political ideology of the left while individualism draws more from the right. However, on a deeper level they share some haunting similarities.

To see them, let's step back a bit. Until now, we have been considering mostly the health problems of the developed world, because biohealth arose from biomedicine and medicalization, both of which had their origins in the developed world of the West. During the period of biomedicine, colonial control of Africa and southern Asia was in its heyday; independence and the beginnings of "development" there occurred during the following period of medicalization. By the end of the 1970s, however, there were some ominous signs that medicalized development may not be as successful in the South as it appeared to be in the industrialized West. The health problems were different, the peoples' cultures were different, and the new countries were still "developing"—or, from the point of view of the West, poor.

The attempted eradication of malaria provides an interesting example.[10] Using extensive biomedical knowledge accrued during the period of biomedicine, the World Health Organization set out to eradicate malaria. It failed in most countries, and when considering why, concluded that the fundamental problem was the distribution of basic health services. To address this problem, the UN convened a conference in Alma Ata, USSR in 1978 to make clear how to confront these problems. The result was the official birth of Primary Health Care (as a system), and the declaration that the world should have "Health For All by the Year 2000." In their Declaration,[11] the fourth of ten statements was this: "The people have the right and duty to participate individually and collectively in the planning and implementation of their health care."

At first glance this appears to be a very progressive notion, a challenge to paternalism and top-down development. It sounds like the 1960s slogan "power to the people." But look more closely. The Declaration, compiled by globalized health experts, spelled out in detail exactly what Primary Health Care (PHC) should be, including the "eight elements" (nutrition, water and sanitation, family planning, etc.) that all PHC programs should address. Though it defines health broadly ("not merely the absence of disease . . ."), it is clear that the wellbeing it seeks should be sought with the tools of Western technology. Though it admits PHC "reflects and evolves from the . . . sociocultural . . . characteristics of the country," it quickly adds that this should be "based on the application of the relevant results of social, biomedical and health services research"—

10. Downing, *Suffering and Healing in America*, chs 12.
11. Declaration of Alma-Ata, 1.

and not, therefore, a local *shalom*. It openly calls for government responsibility in setting up PHC systems, and then stipulates "maximum community and individual self-reliance and participation in the planning, organization, operation and control of primary health care."

Alan Peterson and Deborah Lupton, in their analysis of the new public health, call this "the duty to participate."[12] Their example is the UN Healthy Cities project, especially in Europe, but the principles (and the phrase itself) are drawn from the same WHO thinking we have just looked at, and their critique applies equally to PHC. They point out that the style and substance of community participation is set by experts and involves adhering to an "administrative model of decision making" and an obsession with "enumerating, counting, and calculating." The approach clearly assumes that scientific knowledge is superior to lay knowledge. Participation gives the appearance of community control, but since many of the fundamental reasons for ill health in a community are national or transnational, the activities of local people often end up as "little more than tokenism."[13]

Peterson and Lupton then put these comments into perspective. They show that the growth of the terms "community" and "participation" in the 1970s came "in the context of the state's efforts to reduce the costs of health and welfare services by shifting the burden of responsibility for services from the state onto 'the community.'" This then "served to obscure the return to reliance on the market, on families (particularly women), and on individuals themselves to meet basic needs." It "shifts the blame for problems from individuals onto 'communities.'" Yet those fundamental problems leading to ill health are often neither in the control of individuals nor local communities. They are "broader issues such as regional disparities in wealth, trade imbalances, militarism, racism, unemployment, exploitative work practices, and indeed problems inherent in the Western model of development."

We are back to where we started five paragraphs ago. On the surface, community participation is the opposite of individual responsibility. But for biohealth, they function exactly the same way. Biohealth skillfully directs our attention away from the fundamental causes of ill health—disparities in wealth, trade imbalances, and the rest—and tells

12. Peterson and Lupton, *New Public Health*, chapter 6.

13. See also Downing, *Wedding Goes On Without*, chapter 4 "Community Health" for an example.

us as individuals or communities that it's up to us. It is an understandable strategy: biohealth relies on multi-microscopic evidence, and there is plenty of evidence to prove that people and communities that change their behaviors will be a little "healthier." But biohealth is also part of the technological system, a system that is not interested in addressing disparities in wealth, trade imbalances, and so on because it is the system that creates them.

This observation, that the fundamental causes of ill health are not under our control as individuals or communities, is neither new nor esoteric. We saw earlier, at the end of the medicalization chapter, that a purely biomedical view of disease causation is too narrow, and that this was recognized nearly two hundred years ago in Europe. Nortin Hadler estimates that 75 percent of ill health and premature death in the US today is linked with lower socio-economic status; only 25 percent is due to our individual behaviors.[14]

But it is still very tempting to focus on those obvious behavior patterns that affect health, behaviors that appear subject to change. The child that does not sleep under a mosquito net will more likely get malaria. The community with few latrines or an unprotected water source will have more people with diarrhea. The individual who smokes will get emphysema. The community without access to Pap smear screening will have more women with cervical cancer. All this is true. But if Hadler's statistics are representative, that means all of our preventive efforts ignore 75 percent of the problem—issues such as why some communities still have endemic malaria, and why cigarettes are made in the first place. When individual responsibility and community participation are successful—and we have evidence to demonstrate their success—we have addressed only 25 percent of the causes of ill health.

As citizens of the realm of biohealth, we live in this 25 percent. My training as a doctor—even one interested in prevention—focuses on the 25 percent. It was for this reason that when I first read Ivan Illich's provocative article "Heath as One's Own Responsibility—No Thank You!"[15] I felt like he had overstated. It is at least my responsibility, I felt, to not smoke, to not overeat, to exercise, to wear my seatbelt, and all the rest, even if I can't touch wealth inequities and trade imbalances. How

14. Hadler, *Last Well Person*, 11–12.
15. Illich, "Heath as One's Own Responsibility."

could these personal behaviors not be my responsibility? Then I read the article again, and again and again.

At core, I think Illich's argument is really very simple, and he is clearly talking about Hadler's 75 percent. I cannot be responsible for that over which I have no control. This reflects the truism that every manager knows: responsibility without authority is untenable. Elsewhere Illich says that responsibility is "the soft underbelly of fantasies about power," talking here about people who see extreme poverty in third world countries and feel somehow responsible to "change the rest of the world." But it is mainly people from rich countries who maintain these "fantasies of power" that lead to a sense of responsibility, people from the period (1950–80) that was "subject to planning, designing, and policy-making." However, by 1999 Illich could say that this "organization of power prevalent between 1950 and 1980 has no hold on reality any more."[16]

Once again, 1980—but this time to show us a characteristic of biohealth in silhouette. Biohealth, beginning around 1980, began openly proclaiming that we must take responsibility for our own health. Illich said that by 1980 it became clear that we could *not* take responsibility for things over which we had no control, including the fundamental causes of ill health. When something that a regime wants—such as individuals taking control of their own health—is no longer possible, that is precisely when that regime must proclaim that requirement. When everyone already knows and is doing something, there is no need to advertise it.

Illich's article on personal responsibility for heath provides a more direct view of this post-1980 regime. He begins by reviewing several characteristics (of what I am calling biohealth) that might lead people to think that health cannot be their own responsibility. First, in the regime of biohealth, all care for illness as well as the promotion of health must be done by experts. (He calls this "arrogant disempowerment" due to "professional paternalism.") Second, because of this "requirement," there is a scarcity of experts to provide all the illness care and health promotion needed. (To this he points out that "Today, people are dying of hunger, not from a lack of medicine or surgical interventions.") Third, since we are all part of a system, it is the system's job to auto-correct the causes of ill health. (But the best the system can do, he says, is to provide

16. Illich, *Rivers North of the Future*, 220.

more techniques to deal with the negative side effects of techniques, all amounting to "the management of poisonous systems."[17])

In short, none of these are his reasons for disowning responsibility for his own health. He does not deny responsibility for his own health because it is someone else's responsibility—the experts, the system—but rather because the very concept of responsibility in today's world, he says, is an "illusion." To enter into his thinking a bit more deeply we can return to Hadler's 25–75 percent, and to the Alma Ata Primary Health Care dream.

In 1978 the conveners of the Alma Ata conference rightly saw that disease causation was far broader than individual germs or genes. In seeing disease and health in a much larger context, they began to enter into the 75 percent that shows up as "socio-economic status," and that comes from disparities in wealth, trade imbalances, militarism, racism, and all the rest. However, their approach was "the duty to participate," an approach that planted them squarely in the 25 percent of changeable individual and community behaviors.

Unfortunately, changing the 25 percent behaviors is not very successful if the 75 percent issues are not addressed.[18] In addition, many of those 25 percent "lifestyle" behaviors are directly related to the 75 percent underlying reasons, as we saw at the end of the last chapter. I may choose today to have oatmeal instead of Frosted Flakes for breakfast (if I live in Texas), or sleep under an insecticide-impregnated mosquito net (if I live in Tanzania). But Frosted Flakes are more visible than oatmeal in supermarkets, and the local market may increase the price of insecticide beyond my means. Our 25 percent behavior change always depends on the 75 percent. Illich simply refused the illusion that they were separate.

To conclude, let us return briefly to John Knowles. Two years after he threw down the gauntlet of individual responsibility for health, he was dead—of pancreatic cancer. That is a disease that has some "risk factors"— lifestyle correlates—but they are weak. We don't know why most people get pancreatic cancer, but for many of them it seems to have nothing to do with their lifestyle. Clearly good health is not always in our control; clearly we can't always be held responsible for our health. John Knowles' death proclaimed that as important as our individual choices are, they are not the whole story. His own death metaphorically proved him wrong.

17. Illich, "Heath as One's Own Responsibility," 2–3.
18. Lantz et al., "Socioeconomic Factors, Health Behaviors, and Mortality," 1703–8.

9

Bioethics

IN 2002, A MEDICAL ethics journal (*Cambridge Quarterly of Healthcare Ethics*) published a series of brief articles by some scholars who had been involved with the birth of bioethics thirty years earlier. Though ethical reflection on medicine dates to antiquity, and received more recent publicity in the Doctors Trial in Nuremburg after World War II, the term "bioethics" was first used in the early 1970s. We previously considered how the legal case about Karen Quinlan's fate fueled the public debate in 1976, and how by 1980 bioethics was a fixture of biomedicine. There were several obvious outcomes then for the new regime of bio-health: doctors became more aware of their profession's paternalism; medical research became more aware of its duties to inform and respect its subjects; questions about when to "pull the plug" on folks such as Karen Quinlan became more public as there were more plugs to pull; and philosophers suddenly found themselves being paid to philosophize as medical institutions began hiring medical ethicists.[1]

Ivan Illich, however, apparently did not see the growth of bioethics so positively. He once referred to his book *Medical Nemesis*, published in 1975, as "the appropriate antidote to the emerging epidemic of bioethics."[2] In another context, meeting with 120 bioethicists in Illinois in 1987, he co-authored a statement entitled "Medical Ethics: A Call to De-bunk Bio-ethics,"[3] and ten years later at State College, Pennsylvania,

---

1. See also Toulmin, "How Medicine Saved the Life of Ethics," 736–50.
2. Illich, "Pathogenesis, Immunity, and the Quality of Public Health," 5th paragraph.
3. Illich, "Medical Ethics," 233.

delivered a lecture entitled "The Immorality of Bioethics."[4] We will look at some of the reasons for his specific grievance with bioethics in the next chapter. But first we must consider more generally the role of bioethics within biohealth, and why it might be an "epidemic."

The author of one of the brief historical articles noted above says that "bioethics really started as an inquiry into the largely uncontrolled practices, habits, and proceedings of the medical structure and profession. In doing this inquiry it had to adopt a position of being neither inside nor outside the activity itself," needing both enough understanding of medicine, but also enough distance, to ask the necessary "troubling and vexing questions." Unfortunately, he says, "today . . . the problem is that ethicists have become to be identified with (and, more disastrously, have begun to identify themselves with) the establishment instead of remaining fence-straddlers . . ."[5] Their position originally may be like that of medical sociologists today—except that sociologists were and still are only "outside the activity itself."

One of those sociologists, William Ray Arney (author of *Medicine and the Management of Living* that we considered in the chapter on Systems), has this to say about the role of bioethics in the context of modern institutions: "I tend to think of bio-ethics not as an attempt to reflect on this in a quasi-moral way but as part of the system of power of medicine. (Ethics popped up in other areas as well at the same time it became popular in medicine. Arco oil company was the first to hire a corporate ethicist in the 1970s. In a big show the ethicist's office was located right next to the CEO's office.) Ethics seems, in most instances, to provide intellectual grounding for questionable actions."[6]

From both medical sociology and medical ethics itself, then, is the haunting suggestion that bioethics may not be purely objective moral reflection on the thorny questions of biomedicine. It may not be, as a general inquiry and a profession, the conscience of biomedicine we assumed it was. Of course there is no single bioethical position on any of the troubling and vexing questions we all struggle with. Nevertheless, the general direction of bioethical inquiry is beginning to follow a pattern. Another bioethicist reflecting on the recent thirty year history wrote this: "Words attributed to Daniel Callahan, perhaps erroneously,

4. Mitcham, "Unexpected Friendship."

5. Loewy, "Bioethics," 392–93.

6. Arney, WR, personal communication, December 31, 2007.

often come to mind: 'Do bioethicists ever say no?' There seems to be an overpowering inclination among bioethicists to propose conclusions that are more likely to please the scientific and business communities than to protect the rights of the weak and powerless."[7]

These ethicists we just quoted, a least, seem disturbed by this trend they have identified. One of the clearest examples of this "intellectual grounding for questionable actions" "more likely to please the scientific and business communities" is the article by Maurizio Mori, "The Twilight of 'Medicine' and the Dawn of 'Health Care': Reflections on Bioethics at the Turn of the Millennium."[8] We consider it in some detail not because it is representative of bioethics as a whole (in fact, it is *not*), but rather because it illustrates how biohealth can co-opt and use bioethics.

Mori, an Italian philosophy professor, begins by summarizing some traditional views of bioethics. Its most ancient roots are in clinical medicine, which has traditionally seen health as a natural state that physicians try to help their patients return to. Twentieth century biomedicine attempts the same: to return ill patients to their "natural" state of health. This "returning" Mori sees as "medical conservatism." Social medicine, on the other hand, especially since the nineteenth century sought to modify the social and environmental causes of illness—those factors that prohibit this natural health—and appears to be more progressive. Both, however, accept that there is a natural state of health, a foundational given, a sort of touchstone.

Mori's view is different. He understands health to be far more plastic. Health to him is not a natural given but something we create with the tools of biomedicine; we use these tools not only to treat disease, but also "to fulfill desires and wants." To Mori, bioethics is not merely "an extension of traditional medical ethics," but "a crucial new *cultural movement* which brings us to redefine... our relationships with health and life." Mori's understanding of health and bioethics are central to the self-understanding of biohealth, and deserve a deeper look.

Before biomedicine developed its techniques in the twentieth century, doctors could only cooperate with and sometimes assist natural healing processes. Nature and health *were* givens that could be assisted, but not fundamentally changed. For example, doctors could encour-

7. O'Rourke, "As Time Goes By," 386.

8. Mori, "Twilight of 'Medicine,'" All Mori quotes are from this article, and all quoted emphasis is in the original.

age adequate diet, exercise, sanitation, and peace of mind to enhance a person's immunity—but it was natural immunity fighting an infection, not medicine. In the 20th century, under the regimes of biomedicine and medicalization, we began to learn how to control nature. Doctors could give medications that could eliminate infections in people, even people with lowered immunity. We also found ways to lower that immunity where it was overactive, as in allergies and auto-immune diseases. We were not cooperating with nature, we were controlling it, fighting against those "natural" processes that resulted in disease.

With biohealth we see a third stage of the development of our relationship with nature. Beyond assisting or even controlling nature, now we are beginning to change nature and natural processes, to *transform* them. Clarke and her colleagues see this as the overarching shift from medicalization to biohealth (which they call biomedicalization). "Such transformations," they say, "range from life after complete heart failure to walking in the absence of leg bones, to giving birth a decade or more after menopause, to the capacity to genetically design life itself," as well as transformations "much less dramatic, such as Botox and laser eye surgery."[9] Mori agrees: "Contemporary health care providers are increasingly aiming at *transforming* biological nature to modify it to satisfy a person's needs and to fulfill her autonomous choices."

Transformation of nature itself is certainly a large step beyond simply controlling it—a new paradigm, Mori rightly calls it. We are not really there yet, though we sometimes act as though we were, and we truly seem to be on the way. Sex change operations are an excellent example that Mori celebrates: people now seem able to choose their sex. In fact, medicine and surgery can at present make a man look and feel like a woman (change the phenotype), but cannot yet change that man's genetic make-up from XY to XX (change the genotype). Likewise the person who has "life after complete heart failure" may be alive, but that life is precarious. Botox is successful in removing wrinkles, but is temporary. In many ways we are still functioning in an advanced biomedical and medicalized paradigm, but one that already looks like we are transforming nature. Mori admits that we are at the twilight of the old paradigm and the dawn of the new one.

How far we will move, and how fast, is still unknown. Nevertheless, we have begun to *think* differently about our relationship to natural

9. Clarke et al., "Biomedicalization" 165.

givens, and to function as if our extensive control of nature was fully transforming it, as it already does in small ways. This new sort of thinking *is* Mori's bioethics, and is at the heart of biohealth, which Mori shows by describing its impact on us at the conceptual, individual, and social levels. Reviewing this impact provides an excellent summary of the four characteristics of biohealth we have been considering.

First, systems. Medical ethics was originally derived from reflection on the relationship between patients and their individual doctors. Now, says Mori, "we are passing from an 'artisan medicine' (or 'craftsmanly medicine') to an 'industrial health care system' which has a greater impact on society at large and involves new levels of human interaction." This system, as we saw a few chapters back, is far more complex, and involves contributions from many different professionals. Medical ethics based on the sanctity (or at least respect) of the doctor-patient relationship alone is not sufficient for today's *system* of health care. That is why Mori sees bioethics—the ethics of health care systems—as fundamentally different from medical ethics.

Second, commodities: Mori openly admits that "if the living process is modifiable and manipulable, then health is no longer dependent on the whims of nature, but can be purchased like any other human goods or commodities." Traditional medical ethicists may worry about this "commercialization of the body," but Mori does not. Responding to the "deep and widespread qualm" that "a visit to a 'health-house' won't be much different from a trip to the supermarket" with health providers primarily interested in increasing their profit, Mori suggests that this is simply a matter of health care justice. This is different, he says, from a matter of medical morality. To Mori, the problem is not in making health a commodity, but simply the selfishness of the provider; the only thing needed is proper controls of those who sell it.

Third, considering risk, Mori introduces the term "predictive medicine." We are entering the era, he says, when "we can confidently predict nature's course of action," and consequently will be able to develop a "reasonable control over risks and inconveniences." Predictive medicine has the same foundation as risk analysis: we make predictions based on multiple careful observations of similar phenomena, and of an understanding of the underlying biological processes. And predictive medicine will have an accuracy like that of risk, giving us a percent chance that a certain phenomenon will occur. Predictive medicine, it seems to me, will be just as seductive as risk management.

Finally, Mori closes the loop in this system of health care and makes the connection between predictive medicine and responsibility. When doctors are able to predict a certain occurrence, they are deemed responsible to do something about the yet-to-happen event. However, "we are passing from a sort of 'medical aristocracy' to some kind of 'health care democracy'"—meaning that medical knowledge will be more and more available to patients and potential patients. Mori then predicts that as this knowledge diffuses, as for example with "self-diagnostic machines," "each one of us will become more and more responsible for our own health."

That, then, is a bioethical apologetic for biohealth; it is a defense, not a critique. It asks no "troubling and vexing questions" of biohealth. Instead, Mori suggests we change the name of our enterprise from "medicine" to "health care" (as in his title) to reflect the paradigm change: "Traditional 'medical treatments' (performed to restore health to a natural given) are radically different from new 'health care treatments' (performed to fulfill desires concerning the biological aspects of life)." For Mori, bioethics should not challenge this change, but facilitate it. "We should," he writes, "be willing to change our values and norms in order to adjust to the new circumstances."

Clearly Mori does not speak for all bioethicists; the foundation of his argument is to refute some of their views. In fact some bioethicists, as we saw above, feel that bioethical inquiry should remain enough outside both biohealth and the business community to be able "to protect the rights of the weak and powerless"—even, one supposes, if that means challenging some of the aspects of biohealth. But is that really possible, especially when bioethicists are hired by healthcare institutions? And if a bioethicist did "say no," who would listen?

It is perhaps easier for bioethics to either defend biohealth, as Mori does; or to deal with a discrete set of issues enclosed by biohealth, "issues such as individual autonomy, confidentiality, rights and protections in high-tech medicine . . ." This focus, says Nikolas Rose, means that bioethicists "seldom address the ethical issues raised by the mundane, routine, global depredations of illness and premature death. . . . Why," he asks, "should the 'dignity' of the person at the end of life be a bioethical issue, but not the massive 'letting die' of millions of children under five each year from preventable causes?"[10]

Of course the massive 'letting die' *is* an ethical issue; it comes under the fourth principle (for those who accept the four principles) of distributive justice. We in biohealth and bioethics ignore problems like this for several pedestrian reasons. First, because biomedical institutions hire bioethicists, those institutions decide what questions to ask; they set the agenda. Rose gives an example: "As biotech companies seek to commoditize DNA sequences, tissues, stem cells, skin, cord blood and more, it is clear that 'ethics' has a crucial function in market creation. Products that do not come with appropriate ethical guarantees, notably assurances as to 'informed consent' of donors, will not find it easy to travel around the circuits of biocapital." If biotech companies hire ethicists to ensure ethical rules are followed, it is unlikely those ethicists will question the entire endeavor.

Second, when ethicists do raise troubling searching questions, especially from non-commercial stances such as universities or the UN, what sort of power lies behind their recommendations? Who listens? In-vitro fertilization, a procedure with its own set of ethical questions, has now brought with it the ability to diagnose conditions in the embryo before it is implanted in the uterus. This is called preimplantation genetic diagnosis (PGD). Realizing the additional ethical questions that would arise with this technique, the International Bioethics Committee of UNESCO issued a recommendation that "PGD be limited to medical indications. Therefore sex selection for non-medical reasons is to be considered unethical."[11] The recommendation may be very sensible with a strong moral foundation, but as long as there are people who want to choose the sex of their child and medical providers willing to comply, the recommendation will be ignored.

Finally, it is clear that "massive letting die" is fundamentally a political and economic issue. A member of the International Bioethics Committee just mentioned writes this: "The idea that the combination of scientific progress and free market would spontaneously extend its benefits worldwide, which was dominant in the past two decades, has failed . . . Unfortunately, the undesired but foreseeable result of medical progress tends to increase inequalities, because it is oriented by vested

---

10. Rose, "Molecular Biopolitics," 3–29.

11. Berlinguer, "Bioethics, Health, and Inequality," 1086–91.

interests and directed towards the rich instead of general goals." One example is the "10/90 gap": only 10 percent of the world's health research budget focuses on 90 percent of the world's health problems, mostly problems of poor places. Another example is the functioning policy that has prevailed throughout the world since the late 1980s: "The idea of the priority of primary health care and of the prevention accessible to everybody has been supplanted by high technologies, even in countries where the resources are minimal."[12] Our collective choices of how and where we spend our money are behind why so many poor people die from preventable causes.

Of course this situation is unethical in the sense that it *ought not* to happen. But its causes are political and economic, not inadequate ethical reflection. What difference would it make for bioethicists to enter the fray? Nikolas Rose, in fact, asks an even more probing question: "What forms of expertise does bioethics claim or is it ascribed to support its authority?"—suggesting "it is time to open this peculiar persuasion of bioethics to critical investigation."[13]

Perhaps someone should—remembering that biomedicine does bring with it huge dilemmas and contradictions, and that bioethics has committed itself to walking through that maze with us, doggedly turning over every stone along the way. But whether we praise bioethics or pillory it, we must remember the central role it plays in biohealth. It is true that biohealth can use bioethics as its press secretary, as we have just seen; it is today more "inside" than "outside the activity" of biohealth. But biohealth embraces all biological techniques to produce health, and all of the discourse on them. Even medical sociology, with its more critical "outside" view, can end up advertising for biohealth. Clarke et al, in their penetrating overview of biomedicalization, admit that "our project here cannot help but constitute and promote biomedicalization."[14]

Said differently, biohealth as a complex system is very resilient, one that absorbs and very effectively silences critiques.

12. Berlinguer, "Bioethics, Health, and Inequality," 1086–91.

13. Rose, "Molecular Biopolitics," 3–29.

14. Clarke et al., "Biomedicalization," 184.

10

Life

I AM INTRIGUED THAT EVANGELICAL Christians, especially in the United States, have chosen abortion as their flagship political issue during this period of biohealth. Their "pro-life" position gives us a different window into biohealth, and introduces the final characteristic of biohealth we will consider: how it redefines life.

The origin of the modern pro-life movement is the US Supreme Court decision in 1973 (Roe v. Wade) that had the effect of legalizing abortion across the US. The timing is interesting: this decision came during the period we have defined as medicalization, when problems of all sorts were seen to have medical solutions that we could control. The problem here was an unwanted pregnancy; the solution was a medical procedure to remove the problem. Clearly the procedure did not arise from this period, nor even its ability to be performed safely. What occurred was its legal legitimation, and consequently a great increase in its frequency.

But this was not only, or even primarily, a matter of medicalization. The Supreme Court decision mentioned medical issues, but focused far more on the Fourteenth Amendment's guarantee of privacy for the individual. This decision fit with society's increasing emphasis on individualism and autonomy that we discussed in the chapter on responsibility. Yet it did not ignore the context of this individual privacy: the life of the fetus or potential life within the womb were mentioned more often than the life of the mother. The majority opinion, however, felt that "the potentiality of human life" or the alive fetus were not "persons" according to the Constitution, and therefore not subject to the Fourteenth Amendment guarantees. They considered this together with the nature of abortion laws throughout history—which generally made a distinction between abortion done before quickening and after—and concluded that laws prohibiting abortion in the first trimester were unconstitutional.[1]

This of course was a legal decision, not a moral one—it is vital to remember the difference: the Supreme Court did not declare abortion "moral" any more than it declared physician advertising ethical nine years later. But Evangelical Christians and Catholics felt the legal decision about abortion had immense moral significance. To them, liberalized abortion laws devalued life itself. Our society had again made a move toward controlling or preventing life, as it had done when eugenics was popular in the 1920s and 30s. Then, the Protestant church did not protest and Catholic opposition was muted.[2] Now, however, a renewed religious community decided to draw a line in the sand—only to them it was not in the sand. Abortion was murder, they felt, and a society that allowed any form of murder had lost its moral moorings. Religious pro-lifers determined to re-anchor society onto a respect for life.

Their analysis was sharp and their goal laudable: something had gone horribly wrong in a society that seeks to control its most precious and enigmatic life-gifts. When nine-tenths of Downs Syndrome babies are never born, when healthy life is something that depends on the medical system, when suffering is something we seek to eliminate instead of endure, when deviance is either incarcerated or medicated, when old age is garaged instead of celebrated, when death is fought against instead of embraced . . . all of these characteristics of biohealth proclaim that something has gone wrong with our understanding of what we've decided are the rough edges of life. And for pro-lifers, a re-orienting of our respect for life needed to start at the very beginning.

Now when a pro-life movement exposes society as having a selective and limited understanding of life in all these areas, thereby exposing its thinly veiled anti-life core, that movement is prophetic. Indeed, from the early 1980s there have been small groups of religious pro-lifers (such as Pro-Lifers for Survival and The Seamless Garment Network) who saw the problem in it's entirety, seeking to expose the anti-life bent woven throughout all of modern society. Their focus was not only abortion,

---

1. Roe v. Wade, 1973, IX A.

2. Hall, *Conceiving Parenthood*, ch. 3. For a significant exception, see Chesterton, *Eugenics and Other Evils*.

but also euthanasia, the arms race, war, poverty, the death penalty, and racism: all indications of modern society's loss of respect for life. And curiously, while there is biblical rationale for all of these issues, the largest volume of biblical texts concerns poverty and justice, not abortion.

These groups, however, had essentially no political impact; US election issues have remained stuck as pro-life (= there should be a law against abortion) vs. pro-choice (= there shouldn't be). The exposure of society's anti-life nature has become mired in a legal battle which reflects the stunted understanding of pro-life as simply anti-abortion. But how did that happen? How did this sincere principled movement become so limited? There are undoubtedly practical reasons: to be effective, a movement must be focused. To join media discussions, we must speak in sound-bites. The danger of this, of course, is that we begin to think in sound-bites, that we forget the context of our advocacy. But there is a deeper reason for the narrow focus on abortion, and it opens the matter of how biohealth has redefined life.

Simply stated, "life" has a very different meaning today than it has had throughout most of history. In the Genesis account of the origin of the world, nature itself was alive: the earth produced vegetation and animals, the sea itself brought forth fish. That concept of nature being alive remained in place in Western thought throughout the Middle Ages—until the Renaissance. Then, as the scientific revolution unfolded, people began to understand *how* things worked in nature, and in the process discovered that nature itself wasn't alive, only certain things in nature were alive. This analytical approach helped people increase their control and use (and abuse) of nature and natural resources.[3] By the beginning of the nineteenth century, biology ("the science of life") was born, and scientists set out to determine exactly what separated inorganic matter from living things.[4] They eventually called the essence of life "protoplasm"; today we call that essence DNA.

In many senses, of course, modern science is far more "accurate" than Genesis or Middle Age thinking—and this scientific accuracy is what enables biomedicine to develop such control over disease and life processes. But this accuracy comes with a cost: the more focused our definition of life is, the more limited it becomes. There is some value in calling the earth "alive" because it does bring forth trees and insects

3. Merchant, *Death of Nature.*
4. Illich, "Brave New Biocracy."

and birds in a parallel way that a mother brings forth a child. When we become scientifically accurate and point out that really it is nitrogen in the soil and carbon dioxide in the air (not themselves alive) which enable a seed (alive) to grow into a tree, we inadvertently devalue the earth and atmosphere; we disable the metaphor of the earth as mother of the tree. If the focus is nature as alive, the metaphor works; if the focus is biological life, the metaphor fails.

Coming back to the pro-life movement: at the core of the movement is a recognition that very liberalized abortion policies reflect a flagrant disrespect for life. But in our medicalized society, the definition we use for life is not the larger biblical or Middle Ages definition, but the narrower, more focused scientific definition. The life that we now want respect for is limited to whatever has genetic material—and excludes whatever does not. Now clearly there is significant overlap between the historic definition of life and the scientific one. But it is the areas with no overlap that highlight the problem. In the extreme, we swallow camels and choke on gnats: a pro-lifer has moral difficulty with an IUD as a birth control device because it prevents implantation of a fertilized egg (DNA-containing life), but has less moral difficulty with economic *policies* (without DNA) that enrich the already rich and impoverish the poor, thereby diminishing their life.

Return for a moment to Roe v. Wade. As a legal body, the Court had to deal with the concept of "person" as it appears in the Constitution, written before we had a scientific DNA definition of "life." The Constitution protects the rights of a person, not "a life." Yet in determining that the Constitutional "use of the word [person] is such that it has application only postnatally," the court did not therefore rule that the fetus had no rights. "The pregnant woman," it declared, "cannot be isolated in her privacy. She carries an embryo and, later, a fetus . . . The woman's privacy is no longer sole and any right of privacy she possesses must be measured accordingly."[5] The *legal* decision was to strike down laws prohibiting abortion because they could not be defended *according to the US Constitution*. The moral question of respect for life, and the relationship between "a life" and "a person," remained unanswered.

Now it is clear that a biological definition of life has been solidly with us for over a century. Why, then, the claim in the opening paragraph of this chapter that it is the recent biohealth regime that has caused us to

5. Roe v. Wade, 1973, IX A and B.

redefine life? We began with the abortion debate because it opened the door to a refinement of this biological meaning that appears especially during this period of biohealth. The historian Barbara Duden says that only recently have people been using the phrase "a life"—mostly when referring either to fetuses or dead soldiers (body counts of "lives" lost),[6] both uses beginning in the 1970s. This new terminology does not at first appear troubling. However, seeing its development over the last thirty years or so begins to show how biohealth has redefined life.

The appearance of this redefined life coincided with and was likely carried by the wave of bioethics which swept in around 1980. A scientific, atomized understanding of life fit well with the atomized understanding of society that bioethics was born into. Despite our penchant for systems thinking, we still think as Descartes taught us: we understand those systems to be made up of many small parts—and in the case of bioethics, independent parts. Bioethics began with autonomy (not community) as its first principle; each person was independent of his or her community. But more than that, each person was simply "a life."

Ivan Illich explored this "life" most thoroughly in "Brave New Biocracy: Health Care from Womb to Tomb,"[7] an article worth reviewing at length as it explicitly connects this "life" with several of the characteristics of biohealth we have been describing. Illich confirms the role of bioethics in this new understanding of "a life." He says that personhood, according to bioethics, is rooted in "the 'scientific ability' of bioethicists to determine who is a person and who is not through qualitative evaluation of the fetish, 'a life.' . . . While up to now the law implied that a person was alive, [some bioethicists] demand that we recognize that there is a deep difference between having a life and merely [sic!] being alive." This "act of possession" (having a life) marks "a life" as property, or as a commodity, in much the same way as we found health to be a commodity.

Thinking of these gifts of life and health, these intangibles, as things we can own fundamentally affects our attitude toward them. If life and health are gifts, contingent on the aliveness of nature (or, for Christians, "contingent on the incessant creative will of God"), we cannot posses them as property. We cannot buy or sell them, compete with or for them, or "improve" them as we could a piece of real estate. We do not have this

6. Duden, *Disembodying Women*, 50–55; Duden, "Ivan Illich," 5–6.

7. Illich, "Brave New Biocracy."

much control over life and health, though we presume to. We even countenance a legal term, "wrongful life," that refers to a person that legally should not exist: usually a person born with severe disabilities that could have been diagnosed prenatally and aborted. The term did not appear in the medical literature until 1973, after Roe v. Wade.

In the regime of biohealth, however, "wrongful life" makes sense, because in biohealth we do assume control of both life and health. Because "a life" is a *thing* (Illich calls it a "substantive"—a noun), we treat it like other things. "'A life' is amenable to management, to improvement and to evaluation in a way which is unthinkable when we speak of 'a person.'" We view health the same way: "health as an orienting behavior which requires management . . ." The consequence is clear: if this "life" is a commodity we possess, then we have responsibility for it.

"Physicians are taught today to consider themselves responsible for lives from the moment the egg is fertilized through the time of organ harvest. They have become the socially responsible professional manager not of a patient, but of a life from sperm to worm. Physicians have become the bureaucrats of the brave new biocracy that rules from womb to tomb." But not just physicians: "self-appointed health experts now . . . put the responsibility of suffering onto the sick themselves." Responsibility flows directly from owning something, even if that something is life.

However, as we saw in the chapter on responsibility, Illich himself rejected this responsibility; he said it was an illusion. There is the same sentiment in "Brave New Biocracy," and here he makes explicit the change in his thinking. At the end of the period of medicalization and the dawn of biohealth (1976), Illich published *Medical Nemesis*, the last chapter of which was called "The Recovery of Health." Near the end of that chapter he wrote, "Health designates a process by which each person is responsible . . . . The level of public health corresponds to the degree to which the means and responsibility for coping with illness are distributed among the total population."[8] However, by 1994 (in "Brave New Biocracy") he was writing, "A few decades ago . . . it seemed possible that I could share responsibility for the remaking of this manufactured world. Today, I finally know what powerlessness is. I know that 'responsibility' is an illusion."

8. Illich, *Medical Nemesis*, 273–74.

Finally, we return to systems thinking. In our chapter on systems, we suggested that there was a crucial difference between natural systems (such as the human body or an ecological niche) and technological systems. Illich seems to be referring to this same comparison in "Brave New Biocracy." He mentions ecology as "the study of correlations between living forms and their habitat," and then immediately begins talking about cybernetic systems as "both model and reality." Now the word "cybernetic" can apply to any communication system, whether a natural mammalian nervous system or an electronic internet. However, we have already seen the crucial difference between the two: technological systems must be efficient (not an immediately obvious defining characteristic of natural systems); and technological systems are autonomous, lacking in feedback (a factor always present in natural systems).

Now, when we recognize the parallels that are there between the two sorts of systems, a technological system can become a model for the natural system. However, as Illich says, with systems thinking any cybernetic system becomes "both model and reality." "Within this style of thinking," he continues, "life comes to be equated with the system . . . Being conceived as a system, the cosmos is imagined in analogy to an entity that can be rationally analyzed and managed." In other words, we think of natural systems in the same way as we are used to thinking of technological systems, as systems that we can tweak and control.

What happens when we apply this sort of technological systems thinking to the "system" of life? There are two possible responses. We could recognize the fundamental differences between the two sorts of systems, learning from the models we make but being careful not to collapse the model into the reality. Or . . . we could redefine life as "a life," a technological system, and treat it that way. Illich illustrates this redefinition by re-looking at one of western civilization's origin stories: "In a new kind of reading, Genesis now tells how Adam and Eve were entrusted with life and the further improvement of its quality. This new Adam is potter and nurse of the Golem, his artificial creation." This is the response biohealth has chosen.

Now we have come full circle, but when we return to the beginning and the abortion debate we find a surprise. Pro-lifers have been defending the rights of the fetus on the basis that it is "a life," the very same understanding of life that biohealth has chosen. How did this come about?

For biohealth, the evolution from a historical understanding of life (as part of the aliveness of nature) to the biomedical understanding (as that substance containing DNA that we possess and have responsibility for managing and is part of the system of life) was gradual—and, in retrospect, inevitable. Biohealth is concerned with processes, not persons; with mechanisms, not morality. Considering each human to be "a life" works in this regime, whether we view life as a machine or a system or both. Of course a fetus is a life: it can now be operated on before birth to be repaired; it can likewise be disposed of if repair is felt not to be possible (or if its very existence was a "mistake"). But this is no different from lives after birth: in biohealth they are optimized if nothing is wrong with them, repaired if something is, and (in theory at least) disposed of if they are "wrongful" or if their quality declines beyond bearability.

The process of latching onto "a life" for pro-lifers, however, seems to have been more abrupt. When the US Supreme Court declared in 1973 that a fetus was not a person under the law, those opposed to abortion on moral grounds needed to scramble for a counter argument. The law (and, frankly, common sense) would not allow them to insert personhood into the uterus; but their moral sensitivity (and, frankly, another part of common sense) told them that routinely scooping fetuses out of uteruses for reasons of "choice" betrayed a selfishness that damages society. But they needed an argument more than their moral outrage, and it came easily: "But the fetus is a life!"

Perhaps it came too easily. "The fetus is a life—just like an adult is a life." Without realizing it, they had grasped the reduced biological definition of a life that biohealth had been honing. In being forced to accept that legally fetuses were not persons, they embraced "a life" as that quality which fetuses shared with people already born—and in the process personhood faded for both fetuses and adults. Without meaning to, pro-lifers had made a Faustian deal: they agreed that that the essence of being human was "a life"—a biological life—and that allowed them to call fetuses human. But to do this they had to let go of personhood.

The evidence for this lies not in what they do, but in what they ignore. Their argument that fetuses are alive is compelling, but they remain silent in the face of biohealth's insistence on managing all of our lives. Our personhood is constantly violated, as we saw in the chapter on systems, when biohealth maps out an optimal life trajectory for each of us. As health has become passive—we no longer heal, we are healed by the system—living is also becoming passive. We no longer live, we instead have a life which is managed by experts. And pro-lifers remain silent about this insidious decay of the art of living.

PART III

Biohealth in Action

We have looked in some detail at the history of biohealth, how it emerged from biomedical science and a medicalized society. We have also considered several of its characteristics. But the question lingers: does biohealth really exist? It has no holy book like the Koran, no founder like Marx, no headquarters like the Pentagon, no definitive product like an automobile. Biohealth is more of an adjective than a noun; it is the flavor or temperature of modern biomedicine. It is not a plan or a program, yet it is as real as cold or pink or dry.

As we have tried to show, this biohealth flavor is woven throughout all of biomedicine, all over the world. Nevertheless, there are places where it is concentrated; there are projects and programs that are today inseparable from the biohealth flavor. In this concluding section we will look at two of those places as examples of the impact of biohealth on our lives.

The first is Family Medicine. Though its parent general practice has a very long history—as long as that of medicine itself—Family Medicine is new, not appearing until deep into the medicalization period. It is a very distinct offshoot of general practice, but could not have existed in its current form before biohealth emerged. Chapter 11 will look at Family Medicine's role as the chief contemporary home of biohealth.

Another place where the flavor of biohealth is concentrated is in the management of HIV/AIDS, especially in Africa. AIDS, like contemporary Family Medicine, is a phenomenon only of the period of biohealth, its appearance sandwiched tightly between the election of Reagan and the appearance of the personal computer. Interestingly, the biggest concentration of AIDS is in Africa, the continent least affected by biohealth. Chapter 12 will look at what happens when biohealth invades virgin territory.

Finally, we need to conclude, to ask where all this analysis has brought us. Chapter 13 will take one final look at systems, risk, commodities, and responsibility as the key elements of biohealth, asking to what extent we can embrace the elements of biomedicine apart from the system of biohealth.

11

Family Medicine

AMILY MEDICINE DID NOT begin as a vehicle for biohealth. It was born in the middle of the period of medicalization, a counter-culture response to some of the excesses of that period. It was an intentional attempt to humanize the medical part of the technological society. But biohealth was incubating at the same time—not in opposition to, but as an outgrowth of that same technological society. To see better the interaction between biohealth and Family Medicine, we need to consider the social forces that led to the birth and development of Family Medicine in the West. There were at least four:

1. The most obvious reason for the development of Family Medicine was the growing perception that medicine had become too specialized and fragmented.[1] The expansion of biomedical knowledge meant that no one doctor could master all that knowledge, and increasingly no one tried to. Specialization had become a sort of medicalization of the medical profession itself: the dividing of tasks according to medical knowledge categories, not patient need categories. But as medical tasks were divided, patients felt fragmented. At best, each person in the family had their own doctor; at worst, a given patient might have several doctors. The key Family Medicine values of comprehensiveness and continuity developed as antidotes to this fragmentation.

Those values, at least, are still at the core of Family Medicine. However, such values alone could not defragment the world of specialized biomedicine. I remember the metaphor we were presented with in the 1970s when I was in Family Medicine training. If the specialists with-

---

1. Gutierrez and Scheid, "History of Family Medicine," 7–8.

in medicine were the players in an orchestra, we were to be the orchestra directors: not experts in playing each instrument, but conductors ensuring that all played together smoothly. It was a fine idea—except that it was not a need that the specialists felt, especially for inpatient care. We were ready to conduct, but the symphony was already in process.

We could not force the metaphor, so we changed it. Instead of pursuing a coordinating role in the center of the specialists, Family Medicine in the US moved to the entrance and proclaimed itself gatekeeper. That metaphor stuck: those who financed medical care were pleased with Family Medicine's less technological (and less expensive) management of common acute and chronic problems. Specialists did not complain, because we referred to them patients that really needed their skills. But even more, this form of first contact outpatient primary care was exactly what most European Family Physicians had always done as "GPs."

It was a reasonable compromise. Of all people who report any symptoms in the US, over one third will receive care in an outpatient setting, but only 1 percent will be hospitalized.[2] Family Medicine used this statistic to justify focusing on coordinating outpatient care—and presumably admitting defeat in defragmenting biomedicine at its core.

2. Although this attempt to respond to over-specialization may be the official and specific reason Family Medicine was born, in the US at least, there were other social forces that dovetailed with this. The 1960s was a time of increased social awareness (and tumult), especially among students in the US and Europe. Some who were studying medicine found in Family Medicine a counter-cultural identity, a "movement" that challenged the staid structures and conservative politics that biomedicine had adopted. By 1969 in the US, "family physicians could see themselves as both future participants in a new, well-funded health care mainstream, based on community health . . . and as revolutionaries in the house of medicine, taking on the power of the medical elite."[3]

But counter-culture movements are hard to sustain, especially when the culture being countered is biomedicine. Within a decade, "the image of family medicine leaders as social reformers seeking access to care for all" had been marred. "By the late 1970s, the social tide had turned away from reform toward fiscal and cultural conservatism. Family practice

2. Khan et al., "Future of Family Medicine," S11.

3. Stevens, "TheAmericanization of Family Medicine," 233. See also Gutierrez and Scheid, "History of Family Medicine."

was becoming incorporated into the dominant culture of medicine, to which it was supposedly ideologically opposed."[4] Specialization still reigned, at least in the hospitals, and community health was upstaged by "managed care" in the US. Europe had been far more successful in creating national health systems, and Family Physicians found a natural role as gatekeepers in those systems. But, as in the US, gatekeepers had little influence on what happened inside the gate.

3. A third element, present underneath these influences for the entire second half of the twentieth century, has been a gradual shift in the delivery of biomedicine as it has come to grips with chronic disease. We mentioned at the end of the second chapter that this process began with the isolation of insulin. But how long it has taken biomedicine to adjust gives a clue to the magnitude of the change needed: Fox, as we saw, pinned his entire analysis of the twentieth century disarray of American health policy on its "inattention to the burden of chronic disabling illness."[5]

Even today, the change is not complete. A recent analysis of American Family Medicine points to the same issue: "The problem is that our current process of care is ineffective and obsolete. Why? Because the brief-visit model is an acute care model—whereas today, in addition to acute care, we also provide preventive care and chronic illness management, and we strive to do this using the biopsychosocial model and with a family systems orientation. The brief-visit acute-care model no longer fits these tasks."[6] If our approaches to healthcare delivery have not been solved, at least the task is clear—and Family Medicine embraces this task of chronic disease management and all that goes with it.

4. Finally, influencing the development of Family Medicine— not specifically focused on it originally, but ultimately key to it—was Engel's biopsychosocial model that we have already considered. The author was a psychiatrist, and his proposal was published nearly a decade after Family Medicine was born in the US; clearly the biopsychosocial model did not *cause* the birth of Family Medicine. However, it (and general systems theory of which it was a part) found a welcome home in Family Medicine—and ultimately upstaged the social move-

---

4. Stevens, "Americanization of Family Medicine," 236.

5. Fox, *Power and Illness*, 1.

6. Scherger, "End of the Beginning," 513.

ments that originated Family Medicine. We will examine these last two elements in detail together.

One of the earliest and most complete pictures of this contemporary view of Family Medicine employing the biopsychosocial model to manage all of life as if it was a chronic disease can be found in Arney and Bergen's previously mentioned book *Medicine and the Management of Living*.[7] Ironically, the book names Family Medicine specifically only once or twice, possibly because Family Medicine has no monopoly on the biohealth Arney and Bergen describe, that biohealth having been present throughout all of biomedicine since about 1980. But now, twenty-five years after the book was first published, it sounds like a commentary specifically on contemporary Family Medicine. It is worth looking at this book once again to see how the argument develops.

Arney and Bergen show that in the period of our history leading up to and including biomedicine, doctors viewed disease as a "thing," an entity that entered a person and wreaked havoc there. The medical task, very clear by 1900 in the approach of William Osler, was to describe how that "thing" acted. As the disease was seen to have a life of its own, the role of the patient was only as a repository of the symptoms and signs left by the disease. The patient's own thoughts and feelings were not important to the diagnosis. Society of course felt compassion for those who were ill, especially chronically ill, but that compassion was not related to the medical task of describing and wrestling with the "thing' inside the patient's body, the disease.

However, by around 1950, these two concerns (diagnosis and compassion) began to come together under the aegis of a new understanding of medicine. Gradually, as other fields of inquiry adopted systems thinking, medicine began to do the same. Instead of viewing disease as a thing on its own, it began to view it ecologically; disease was now not an independent entity, but was the interaction of a toxin or germ or insult with a person. The effects could vary from person to person, so doctors now looked not just for signs and symptoms left by the insult, but how the patient was responding.

Systems language describes it this way: "persons" are actually parts of the hierarchy of systems that make up the biosphere. "Below" them in the hierarchy are their own biological subsystems (circulatory, nervous, immune), and below that molecular, genetic, and atomic subsystems.

---

7. Arney and Bergen, *Medicine and the Management of Living*.

Persons themselves, though, are parts of broader supersystems (family, community, culture), and eventually the entire physical environment and biosphere. In this framework, disease is not an independent entity. Rather, it is a perturbation at some part of the hierarchy of systems, an insult, a throwing that part of the system out of balance. The insult may affect a human subsystem—a bacteria entering a wound; or it may enter a supersystem—the massive increase in corn syrup in the US diet around 1980 that we previously mentioned.

In this systems view, the role of the doctor becomes quite different. In the old reckoning, the doctor was in charge, seeking to hunt down and kill the enemy disease. Now, aware of the interrelationship of all things in ecological thinking, the doctor becomes *part of the system*, someone who works by also perturbing the system, hoping to adjust for the original disease-causing perturbation. Therapy is not simply eliminating the disease, but managing it—an awareness necessary to the twentieth century shift from acute to chronic diseases. In some ways, the role of the doctor had been lowered: now no longer commander, but a co-traveler with the patient on a "joint adventure" to live with the chronic disease neither could eliminate.

However, the medical system, represented by the doctor, suffered no real lowering of status or power. As medicine became comfortable with perturbing the system and managing chronic disease, it also realized the possibilities for managing risk—disease that had not occurred yet—and for optimizing the life of everyone. In this "expanded calling," it developed the optimal trajectories for life that we mentioned in the chapter on systems. It developed guidelines for being born, growing, reproducing, aging, and dying—eventually offering us the possibility of even being "better than well."[8] In this context, we see the relevance of Arney and Bergen's sole reference to Family Medicine: "As medicine adopted an ecological orientation, the surgeon who approached the silent patient in a priestly fashion gave way to the family practice specialist surrounded by a well integrated array of other specialists who approached disease with a new kind of 'watchful and armed expectancy,' much as a prison guard, knowing that his own future is tied to the orderly operation of the prison, watches every movement carefully and listens closely for the faintest, most distant sign of disharmony."[9]

8. Elliot, *Better Than Well*.
9. Arney and Bergen, *Medicine and the Management of Living*, 125.

The metaphor is well-chosen. Disease today is not a single outlaw roaming the country-side liable to attack us unexpectedly—after which we must call the sheriff. Disease now is a building full of hundreds of dangerous outlaws, and good prison guards manage the prisoners to ensure "orderly operation of the prison," and by careful surveillance should be able to tell when a riot or jailbreak is imminent. When an outlaw escapes and citizens are attacked, we still call the sheriff—but the attack was not "unexpected," and both citizen and sheriff can blame the prison guard. Or (more kindly) we all sit down together and analyze how the system of outlaw control broke down.

Family Medicine today is far more prison guard than it is sheriff. This change is evident in the documents of the US Future of Family Medicine project. In the first half of this decade, responding to its own adolescent (or was it mid-life?) identity crisis, American Family Medicine embarked on a "Future of Family Medicine" project, attempting to outline direction for the new millennium. The result was a "New Model of Family Medicine,"[10] the characteristics of which are a table of contents for biohealth. Not so coincidentally, the project was funded in part by pharmaceutical companies and their foundations: the financial center of biohealth.

Look, for example, at the "basket of services" in the new model. The list includes over a dozen services that future family doctors will be routinely providing, services that resemble prison guard far more than sheriff. Certainly the "sheriff" services are still present, in the middle of the list—"diagnosis and management of acute injuries and illnesses" and "of chronic diseases." However, "prison guard" services predominate: integration of care, evaluation of risk status, disease prevention, heath promotion, patient education, supportive care, referral services, advocacy, and quality improvement activities.[11]

All of the tasks, whether surveillance or care, are now seen as problems of management. Certainly the huge amounts of *information*, both research information and patient information, require management skills. And of course the *processes* involved in ushering the patient through the "complex web of relationships and services," or of "assessment and improvement of their care," also involve the ability to manage.

10. Green et al., "Task Force 1," S33–S50. Also Khan et al., "Future of Family Medicine."

11. Khan et al., "Future of Family Medicine" S17.

But now the same sorts of skills can be used to manage the *relationship* between the patient and the doctor, as today with chronic and preventive care "a continuous healing relationship is the essence of care."[12]

This reliance on standardized management technology, even for those tasks such as relationship building that rely mostly heavily on individual personality and intuition, identifies the New Model of Family Medicine clearly as part of the technological society we considered at the end of the chapter on systems. "What makes the model new," say the authors of the project, "is that it is centered primarily and explicitly on the needs of the patient, *it incorporates new concepts from industrial engineering and customer service,* and it integrates these needs and concepts into a coherent and comprehensive approach to care."[13] In the realm of biomedicine, the *relationship* between doctors and patients was still part of a natural social system; it was the biomedicine they prescribed that was part of the artificial technological system. Now, both the relationship and the biomedicine itself are products of the technological system. The New Model of Family Medicine is biohealth in action.

Now let us return to the management of information. A pivotal element of the New Model is the use of electronic medical records to document and store information about each patient, and generate information about when screening tests are due for each potential patient. Interfacing with this would be access to the newest information from biomedical research, ensuring that patients are getting state of the art care. But that new information itself needs to be sifted, or managed, using the techniques of evidence based medicine (EBM). The amount of information is so large that electronic management makes complete sense.

But what is the relationship between the mastery of all this information and the achievement of health in our patients—not just statistically significant improvement of health parameters, as in biohealth, but improved well-being as in *shalom* health? Well-being is difficult to measure, so we often accept proxy measures of well being—such as statistically significant improvement of health parameters . . . and after a while we equate the proxy with the real thing. Consider this example:

12. Green et al., "Task Force 1," S42.

13. Khan et al., "Future of Family Medicine," S13, emphasis mine.

In a continuing medical education (CME) module[14] on information mastery I read in 2006, the material was introduced by a case scenario. The patient described was a retired chemist who had had chest pain and, during a visit to the emergency room, was given several new medications on the assumption that the pain was from esophageal reflux. He was now seeing his Family Doctor in follow-up, presenting him with a paper bag full of these medications and a series of questions about them. The doctor emptied the bag onto his desk, and immediately was faced with even more questions that the CME module was intended to address: what might be the interaction between the new medications he was given and his existing ones for stable angina? What is the role of zinc that the ER doctor had prescribed? What was the evidence for diagnosing esophageal reflux clinically—and if further testing was needed, which tests? I was left with the impression that this poor doctor, not having information at his fingertips because he had not yet mastered EBM, had a less than satisfactory visit with his patient.

The scenario could have proceeded differently. The doctor immediately emptied the bag of medicine bottles onto his desk. He didn't need to. He could have begun by engaging the patient in a conversation about the episode of chest pain. How was he feeling now? What did he think the cause was? Did the medicines he got at the ER help? Did he feel he needed more thorough testing? These of course are questions arising from a "patient-centered" approach, and need not be in conflict with an "evidence-based" approach. However, there is an insidious message in having the doctor open the bag first. In a culture where prescription drugs are advertised on television, where doctors spend far more time studying pharmacology than interview technique (and more time studying interview technique than sociology or literature)—where biomedicine has seeped into every area of our lives so that now even health is only biohealth—in that culture we must honor tablets more than talk. We may *want* to be patient-centered, but many of our patients are already evidence-based. We need to open the bag first.

We can, and perhaps we should, bemoan the reduction of therapy to pills, and the reduction of evidence to numbers. But can we do more than bemoan? We live in a technological system, a system that is now almost totally artificial; a system dedicated to efficiency, lacking in feedback loops. Our problem is not that it is a system, but that it is an

---

14. Ebell, "Information Mastery."

artificial system, one that has displaced whatever natural systems we used to be part of. Natural plant and animal systems are fenced off as national parks; natural social systems are overwhelmed by technology. Natural healing systems are lost; the Future of Family Medicine is biohealth's response.

But natural healing systems are not lost everywhere. Biomedicine may have spread throughout the world, but biohealth is still concentrated in the West, where it developed. What happens, then, when biohealth makes a sudden appearance where it has been almost unknown?

12
AIDS In Africa

IT MAY INITIALLY SEEM odd to use the response to AIDS in Africa as a case study for biohealth. AIDS is a single deadly disease; biohealth seems to be about systems management. The largest concentration of AIDS is in the poorest continent; biohealth developed in the richest continents. What is the connection? Perhaps a very brief historical review will set the stage.

AIDS was first described in the United States in 1981—at the very beginning, incidentally, of the regime of biohealth. It was soon found to be prevalent in Africa, especially in Uganda, where the prevalence rose steadily until 1991, and then started falling. The reasons for the rise and fall have been debated, but there is substantial evidence that a main reason for the fall is that people changed their behavior.[1] Uganda was one of the first countries to promote the ABC approach—Abstain, Be faithful to one partner, and use a Condom (in that order), and during the 1980s and early 90s that was their main approach to prevention. Condoms were not widely used, and voluntary counseling and testing (VCT) programs had not yet started. The early fall in Uganda's AIDS prevalence was because of what Ugandans themselves did.

A decade later the zone of highest prevalence had shifted southward, with South Africa now in the spotlight. But during that decade much about AIDS had changed in the West. Testing had improved, and anti-retroviral (ARV) drugs were now available for treatment; an American Family Medicine professor proudly proclaimed to me in 1996 that we had transformed AIDS from a fatal disease to a chronic one. The drugs

---

1. Green, *Rethinking AIDS Prevention*, 11, 141–226.

were readily available in those countries that now carried the pattern of AIDS transmitted among men who had sex with men, and people who used intravenous drugs—now the lesser epidemic. The greater epidemic was in Africa, primarily from heterosexual transmission, but also with an unknown amount of transmission from blood products and unsterile medical needles.[2]

In the 1980s, the West had little to offer Africa to help control its AIDS epidemic—except NGOs with AIDS education programs and, I remember clearly, brand new vehicles bearing the logo of the supporting organization. However, by the end of the 1990s, the picture was very different. The West now had a way to keep people with AIDS alive. It was complicated and expensive using ARV drugs, but it worked—and that's what made the South African story so different from the Uganda story a decade earlier. South Africa was bigger, South Africa had a well-developed activist community from its experience fighting apartheid, but most important was that the West now had drugs to treat what had become a predominantly African disease, but they were too expensive for Africa.

The picture was clear to activists, both in South Africa and in the West: there was a biomedical solution to African AIDS, but it was not available in Africa only because of cost. It was a matter of justice that steps be taken to make the drugs available urgently; every day hundreds of people were dying simply because they lacked those "life-saving" drugs. And the "sides" seemed clear: on the one side was the rich affluent West with powerful pharmaceutical companies refusing to lower their drugs costs, or allow countries like South Africa to manufacture the drugs while they were still under patent. On the other side was a raging AIDS epidemic, unable to afford the drugs.

However, in 2000 yet another "side" developed, and the picture became muddled. Thabo Mbeki, the newly elected successor to Nelson Mandela, became intensely interested in AIDS. The growing epidemic in South Africa had been almost ignored by the government, upstaged by the country's emergence from apartheid, and it was clearly time to wake up. But Mbeki's awakening was not what the activists and the scientists expected—and Mbeki must have known that from the beginning. In early 2000 he wrote a letter to world leaders acknowledging that South

---

2. Gisselquist, "Denialism undermines AIDS prevention," 649–55.

Africa had a major AIDS epidemic, and that it was different from the epidemic in the West.

"It is obvious," he wrote, "that whatever lessons we have to and may draw from the West about the grave issue of HIV-AIDS, a simple super-imposition of Western experience on African reality would be absurd and illogical . . . I am convinced that our urgent task is to respond to the specific threat that faces us as Africans. We will not eschew this obliga-tion in favour of the comfort of the recitation of a catechism that may very well be a correct response to the specific manifestation of AIDS in the West."[3] To Mbeki this was obvious—but it was not obvious to the scientists and activists who saw his approach as an impediment to "roll-ing out" ARV drug programs.

A fight developed between Mbeki and almost everyone else. It was long and acrimonious, and quickly degenerated into an argument about the cause of AIDS. Mbeki attempted to make clear the context of poverty in which AIDS flourished; his opponents accused him, falsely it turns out, of denying the viral cause of AIDS. Eventually Mbeki lost.[4] The result was that the "catechism that may very well be a correct re-sponse to the specific manifestation of AIDS in the West" was in fact "superimpose[ed] on African reality"—and that catechism has a distinct flavor of biohealth.

What makes this story so poignant, and risky, is how rapidly this package of biohealth came to Africa. When I left Kenya in 2001 for three years, ARVs were only available for those who could afford them—very few people indeed. When I returned in 2004 there were in place several massive ARV programs in Kenya alone, a pattern repeated across the continent—and in most programs the ARV drugs were either very in-expensive or free. And the programs were working: death rates of those with AIDS were falling, and early studies of adherence to the drugs showed results equal to, or more often better than, adherence rates in the West. It bears repeating: biomedicine works.

But how is this biomedical intervention an illustration of biohealth? A look at AIDS programs in Africa demonstrates many of the charac-teristics listed in Part II of this book. The foundation of most AIDS programs is VCT—voluntary counseling and testing. This is a classic screening program that assumes everyone in the population is at risk,

3. Mbeki, "Letter to World Leaders," pars. 26–27.

4. Downing, *As They See It*, chapter 3.

and the only way to know for sure who actually has the disease is to test everyone. "Know your status" is now a rallying cry throughout Kenya; it has become a duty, a responsibility, of each citizen to know his or her HIV status. But this is not simply screening: it is "voluntary," meaning the responsibility is individual, not enforced by legal sanction (but rather by social pressure). Furthermore, it comes with counseling, private pre- and post-test counseling to the individual tested (unique, by the way, to HIV testing) ensuring that the person's autonomy is preserved.

Now this screening program is very complete, with training and certification required for anyone involved with the counseling part. The program is also very Western. Planning the future of my health based on risk is a very recent phenomenon even in the West, as we have seen. And grounding a program in individual autonomy is also very Western; traditional African societies are still based in families and communities whose authority is as important as that of the individual. An illustration of this difference is in how many Kenyans confront the "confidentiality" that is such a pivotal part of the counseling: they openly speak of "shared confidentiality," shared with the family members. This modification is a gentle reminder of how Western biohealth can be.

A recent *Guardian Weekly* article highlighted an even more pro-found challenge to screening. The author noted that even though Botswana provided free ARV drugs for all AIDS patients as early as 2001, only 15 percent of the estimated 100,000 people with AIDS had come for treatment—many choosing not even to get tested. "Why," asked the subtitle of the article, "when treatment is freely available, would so many choose not to know if they are HIV positive?" At the end of the article there is a glimpse from Sizwe, a traditional rural South African who has chosen not to get tested. It wasn't just stigma—"that is not the main reason I won't test. . . If I know I am HIV positive, I will no longer be motivated to do the things I am doing now. It will all be meaningless for me . . . If I test positive, I will no longer get up in the morning to work."[5]

This is a startling and poignant window into the reality of life in rural "undeveloped" Africa. Any proponent of biohealth could quickly answer Sizwe: "But drugs are available! You won't die right away, it's no worse than diabetes, many people on drugs are living positively, you shouldn't be depressed, etc., etc." The biohealth message is watertight—and "may very well be a correct response to the specific manifestation of

5. Steinberg, "'Not a Disease you Look For,'" 25–27.

AIDS in the West" where biohealth originated. But Sizwe knows his own family, his own culture, his own life, and he knows how far a biohealth approach is from the life he knows. We can explain to him how he is "wrong"—or we can listen.

The prevention messages that come with this biohealth catechism are also very Western. African approaches, as we have seen, are inclusive: A+B+C. Western approaches often end up being exclusive. We may verbally assent to an ABC approach, but in practice many in the Western public health establishment feel that prevention = condoms. In response, many conservatives have talked of "abstinence only" approaches. ABC in the West has become A vs. C. Benezet Bujo, an African theologian, summarizes the problem: "'If an information campaign is satisfied with advertising condoms, without exposing the deeper causes and ignoring the ethical questions, then one is merely treating the symptoms.' Advertising condoms rather promotes the consumer mentality, reducing sexuality to a commodity . . . Only an ethical conviction is able to fight this consumer mentality efficiently and to restore sexuality its dignity . . . 'Neither purely technical advice (use condoms, prevent AIDS!) nor moral admonitions (remain faithful!) are sufficient to control the disease. The prevention and stopping of AIDS does not depend solely on the individual but on the quality of our institutions, changes in culture, economy and politics as well.'"[6]

Another example of biohealth prevention is the recent research showing less AIDS spread in communities where the men are circumcised. Very likely circumcision makes a "statistically significant difference" in viral transmission. But in Africa circumcision is not just a medical procedure. It is a means of initiation into adult life; it is also a sign of ethnic identity. Ethnic groups that do not circumcise their boys have other methods of initiation, and the lack of circumcision itself then becomes a sign of ethnic identity. But biohealth is not concerned with identity or *meaning*, it is concerned with *evidence*, with what works. Part of the biohealth catechism is now a recommendation that uncircumcised men be circumcised—a recommendation with a small known effect medically, and an unknown effect culturally.

At the beginning of this decade the African theologian Laurenti Magesa, commenting on biohealth's response to AIDS, wrote this: "So Western organizations—religious, governmental and nongovernmen-

6. Bujo, *Ethical Dimension of Community*, 181–95.

tal—are pouring into Africa. They come bearing all sorts of unsolicited gifts and advice. The advice ranges from how to plant trees to how to get married, and even how to bury the dead! You can fill in anything in between. Much of this advice consists of answers to unasked questions."[7] Peter Kanyandago echoes and expands the same sentiment: "Today it is taken for granted that if Africa is to find a solution to the problem of AIDS, and other problems, it must accept aid and medicine from the West. It is presumed that Africa cannot scientifically and economically manage this problem because it is poor, and therefore needs to be assisted." Kanyandago's view is different: "In order to be able to solve their problems, including that of immune deficiency in general and of AIDS in particular, Africa must start by retrieving and defending their cultural identity, by regaining control over their resources, and by instituting processes for reconciliation and healing."[8]

Finally, the drug treatment itself is another chapter right out of biohealth. We have seen that in the early twentieth century biomedicine created an entirely new category of disease: chronic disease requiring management by chronic medication to prevent death. This sort of disease, as we have just seen in the chapter on Family Medicine, requires an ongoing relationship with a health care provider, and even that relationship should be managed. Biohealth assumes these sorts of relationship today—both with a provider and with a drug—making it easy to forget how recently they developed, and how much of the world has not yet embraced this understanding. We can also forget what else is involved in sustaining these relationships: a place to meet, privacy, transportation, uninterrupted availability of the medications, convenient laboratory facilities to monitor the side effects, a way to pay for all of this—and underneath, an understanding and agreement by the patient that the treatment will be life-long and works best when it is never interrupted.

We should not underestimate the magnitude of introducing this sort of disease management suddenly on a large scale. Dr. Joia Mukherjee of Partners in Health calls this a "new paradigm for public health . . . What has succeeded before in public health are answers that are fairly straightforward and one-shot, like vaccination." However, treating AIDS "looks at treatment of a complicated medical disease with a complicated treatment regimen on a public health scale . . . We're talking about the

7. Magesa, *Christian Ethics in Africa*, 112–13.
8. Kanyandago, "AIDS in Africa."

public health treatment of a chronic condition."[9] We are also talking about the wholesale export of biohealth.

Mukherjee's comment begins to show why the AIDS biohealth catechism is not only poignant, but also risky. Biohealth as a technological system is spreading throughout the world in the same way its parent biomedicine already has. The spread of biomedicine has often brought great benefits, but sometimes at the cost of snuffing out indigenous understandings of disease treatment. At best the two systems coexist and people choose one or the other based on which gives them what they need. But, as we have seen, technological systems must grow; they are pulled forward by the technological imperative, and lack the feedback loop that would hold their growth in check. This unchecked growth ultimately leaves no room for natural indigenous healing systems.

Biohealth is a much more recent technological development, and at present remains mostly where biomedicine was developed or has no competition from indigenous healing systems. But biohealth has a different personality than biomedicine: biomedicine can be offered and used (or rejected) piecemeal, but biohealth comes as a package. It self-consciously sees itself as a total system, and its concern is the health of the whole population—a "health" it defines, and then tells the population is their responsibility. It is intimately connected with, and depends on, the commodities that the rest of the technological system produces. Biomedicine may offer us real choices when indigenous healing systems still exist, but biohealth swallows all alternatives (as we've seen with complementary and alternative medicine). Biohealth will ensure that biomedicine has no competition.

Mbeki saw this coming. During an interview on South African television in 2001, he was asked if he would take an AIDS test. He began a rather complicated explanation of the way he was approaching AIDS, saying that "the matter of whether I take an HIV test or not, I think is irrelevant to the matter. It might be dramatic, and make newspaper headlines . . ." But here the interviewer interrupted him: "But would it not set an example—the president takes an AIDS test?" Then Mbeki responded, "No, but it would be setting an example within the context of a particular paradigm . . . "[10] The world media had decided inaccurately that Mbeki did not believe that HIV caused AIDS; they probably assumed this com-

9. Quoted in D'Adesky, Moving Mountains, 107.

10. Mbeki, interview with Debra Patta.

ment about paradigms referred to the biomedical paradigm vs. the dissident paradigm, the one that did not believe HIV caused AIDS. But more likely Mbeki was referring here to the biohealth paradigm that was invading Africa; the catechism that was designed in and for the West.

Mbeki, of course, was not alone, despite the impression left by the media. He was reflecting a widespread frustration in Africa at Western hegemony,[11] seen in the comments by Magesa and Kanyandago above. But more than this, Mbeki was critiquing one "particular paradigm" (biohealth) from the foundation of another—African healing wisdom. In that paradigm, the health of an individual could not be separated from the health of a community.[12] In "the African concept of health," says Emmanuel Katongole, "individuals could only be considered healthy if they belong to a healthy community. Conversely, because a deep spiritual and religious conception of the universe generally characterizes life in Africa, it follows that health and sickness in Africa are never regarded as merely physical or biological. These are at once social, somatic, religious and spiritual phenomena," pointing to "a holistic vision of well-being and flourishing, which, according to the biblical tradition, is God's *shalom.*"[13]

Mbeki could see that the Western catechism of AIDS control was rooted in a paradigm quite different from the one he grew up in; that even without that catechism, there was something at work in Africa, something that could be built on. But to the Western proponents of the biohealth paradigm, there was *nothing* in Africa: a medical approach for AIDS needed to be introduced. An African proverb says "A foreigner sees only what he already knows." The foreigners who created and introduced a biohealth approach to AIDS had already lost any sense of *shalom* health. They could only see in Africa what they already knew, and so could not see *anything.* It was up to them to rescue Africa.

The rescue package was immense: $15 billion in 2003 for the first five years *just* from the Bush government, supplementing billions from the UN Global Fund and private foundations. Five years later the US tripled their commitment. Since they saw *nothing,* they decided to build from the ground up. And in one sense, there was "nothing": biohealth

11. See, for example, Achebe et al., *Beyond Hunger in Africa,* 3–8; and Mudimbe, *Invention of Africa,* 15.

12. See Armah, *Healers.*

13. Katongole, "Age of Miraculous Medicines," 111.

had not made a foothold in rural Africa. Chronic disease and all that was involved in treating it—regular supplies of medication, habits to take the medicine, clinics to be seen in, laboratories to test for side effects, money for regular transport—all of these were sparse. The West had once again found virgin territory to colonize.

But what would have happened if Mbeki had had a chance to develop his approach, "to respond to the specific threat that faces us as Africans," to work within the other paradigms he must have had in mind when he declined to publicly take an HIV test? How might things have turned out if instead of ridiculing Mbeki, the media had, if not welcomed his approach, at least tried to understand him? Why was there no attempt to involve the scholarship (some of which we have drawn from in this study) that agreed with much of Mbeki's critique while still affirming (as did Mbeki) the role of the HIV virus in the AIDS epidemic? How might medical care throughout the world have benefited if South Africa had developed care for AIDS rooted in the African concept of health that Katongole described above—care that undoubtedly would have involved ARVs? If, in other words, African *shalom* had driven the process instead of biohealth?

We will never know. African healing wisdom of course is still present in people and families in rural communities where biohealth has not yet fully penetrated; it's imprint is still recognizable in urban people who will be buried in the village of their ancestors. But the opportunity to preserve some of this African *shalom* corporately in the response to a major new disease is lost. Maybe it is not possible to truly blend a natural system with an artificial one; maybe, as Ellul reminded us, artificial systems are "given to pure growth" and will inevitably consume or mow down everything in their path.

POSTSCRIPT 2008: The fall from power of both Mbeki and Bush in the same year generated a review of their roles in the events surrounding AIDS at the beginning of the decade. Two parallel themes emerged: how could such a brilliant leader like Mbeki be so wrong about AIDS? And how could Bush, who seemed to get everything wrong from Iraq to Katrina to the economy, get it so right about AIDS? These puzzling questions betray a deep-seated unconscious commitment to the regime of biohealth. For those who assume that the route to health is via the biomedical sciences, Mbeki's stance was unconscionable, and Bush's exemplary.

However, it is only our passionate belief in biohealth that blinds us. If we instead remember that health is wholeness, that individuals can only be truly healthy if they belong to healthy communities, that *shalom* health is as much political and economic and spiritual as it is biological—if we accept this understanding of health, the confusion about Mbeki and Bush begins to clear. Both men were in fact consistent with themselves: Mbeki continued to raise the hard questions about conventional wisdom that he cut his teeth on in the antiapartheid struggle; Bush continued to promote, for every problem, the free market solutions he cut *his* teeth on in oil. Mbeki found himself on the wrong side of those with financial power (the media, pharmaceutical interests), and was crucified. Bush provided a $15 billion windfall, over half going to one of the most profitable industries in the world—and he found a legacy for his failed presidency.

We cannot rewrite this chapter of biohealth. The best thing we can do is mourn.[14]

14. Downing, *As They See It*, 168–74.

13

Conclusion

A T THE BEGINNING OF this book I said that biohealth was antihealth. This is a profound irony, as biohealth grows out of biomedicine, and biomedicine very effectively eliminates, cures, manages, or prevents so many diseases that attack our health. Let us look again at the foundations of biomedicine.

The success and power of biomedicine are rooted in a combination of two quite different approaches. The first is Cartesian—looking at the smallest parts of something living to discover how it works, and how to fix it when it breaks. This approach dissects and separates, moving in the opposite direction from wholism/health. The other approach is epidemiologic—looking at human disease in the aggregate, the largest part possible, both to discover new patterns and to test new interventions. This gives a "whole" picture, but one based only on probability, and therefore sometimes irrelevant to the individual.

Either approach alone can give us tools: Banting and Best isolated insulin by looking only at the pancreas; John Snow discovered the source of cholera in London by reviewing maps and numbers of people with cholera. The first approach dates to the middle of the seventeenth century, the second two hundred years later. Both are pivotal in contemporary medical research: the first is at the core of genetic research, the second the foundation of contemporary evidence-based medicine (EBM). Both continue to give us tools that "work," that provide statistically significant improvements in whatever it is we want to improve.

But this power, this success, has not gone unchallenged. James Le Fanu, as we have seen, suggests that these two approaches are dead ends, that they signal the fall of modern medicine.[1] Ivan Illich, on the other hand, did not question the existence of the power. He saw the tools resulting from these two approaches to be powerful enough to create negative side effects, which he said were counterproductive, canceling the benefits of that power; he called that process medicalization.[2] Though Le Fanu and Illich come to opposite conclusions—one says biomedicine has lost its power, the other that its power is magnified and dangerous—both join those[3] who challenge the common assumption that biomedicine is what makes and keeps us healthy.

One or both of these challenges could of course be misdirected. But throughout this book we have tried to gather stories, opinion, and evidence that suggest that biomedicine is not the essence of our *health*. It's power (even if Le Fanu is right and that power is fading) is real enough, and can undoubtedly change the course of many diseases. The open question is not the *power* of biomedicine, but its *goodness*, its *necessity*—and certainly its relation to health. Biomedicine, wearing the garb of biohealth, is our health emperor, but are we deceived enough to think the emperor is lavishly dressed?

Many of us are. Lee Hoinacki, a close friend of Ivan Illich, paints a troubling picture of what we've called biohealth as a religion, "a new international church."[4] Like all religions, this one grew in a particular place ("the North") among a particular group of devotees ("privileged persons . . . with more education and access to information"). These disciples seek "to be treated in up-to-date cathedrals of care" and "worship an abstraction, health." "They believe, they have a religious faith in the scientific-technological medical system as the principal means to obtain health." In fact, members of this religion adhere to a "mostly unquestioned faith in the principle propositions of the creed," language strikingly similar to Mbeki's reference to the "comfort of the recitation of a catechism" that he saw located in the same place as Hoinacki's "new international church," the developed West.

---

1. Le Fanu, *Rise and Fall of Modern Medicine,* 239, 339.

2. Illich, *Medical Nemesis,* Part II and chapter 6.

3. For example, Dubos, *Mirage of Health* and McKeown, *Role of Medicine.*

4. Hoinacki, *Dying Is Not Death.* All quotes in this and the following 5 paragraphs are from 145–46. There is a similar image in Mendelsohn's earlier *Confessions of a Medical Heretic,* 17ff., referring to "the Church of Modern Medicine."

There are other characteristics that identify this new religion as biohealth. The followers "supplement [their] obeisance with occasional recourse to so-called alternative medicine"—which, as we have seen, is permitted by the religion. They also, "those who bow before the idol, health . . . assist the medical system to achieve its presumed ends" by how they eat and exercise and live. Their choices of how to live, of course, "are derived from the science and practice of medicine, currently exercised in such acts of faith as regular check-ups and tests for the early detection of cancer and other threats to health."

Most of these faithful never went forward at a biohealth crusade; they were either baptized as infants or started going to this "church" because everyone else did. As with any religion, the priests really believe, and the followers follow. But biohealth, like most secular religions, doesn't really care about meaning or values or personal beliefs (the faith, Hoinacki says, is "mostly unquestioned" anyway). It is satisfied when priests submit to evidence, and when disciples follow its Ten Commandments—one of which is to buy its commodities. As long as you show up and buy, you retain membership. If you don't show up and buy, you're seen as a backslider, but still assumed to be a member.

However, choosing to openly leave the fold reveals another nature of the Church of Biohealth, that of a religious cult. People who deny that health is a god, that medicines are a eucharist, and that regular check-ups are an obligation are treated with incredulity or scorn. If they are powerful enough to possibly influence other believers, they can even be crucified, as Mbeki found out. This is a kind of church that in another age might have pursued a violent Crusade against infidels, but today is more likely to implant computer chips—voluntarily, of course—in people's wrists (or foreheads) that could store their genome and health histories. Keeping those chips updated would give them ready access to the latest offerings of biohealth; not having the chips would make it very difficult to obtain even basic medicines.

Now the zealots of this religion of biohealth are, Hoinacki tells us, "the apparently favored ones of our world." But they "present a great stumbling block to the ordinary person's need to live, not a religious, but a human life." When health becomes organized as a religion, a religion as jealous and controlling as we just saw, it invades our freedom. "The planners and designers of most institutions attempt to make them as regularized and efficient as possible: they want to create systems."

These systems, which began with "privileged persons" in the North, are rapidly spreading worldwide. "I am tempted," Hoinacki continues, "to conceive of and order my life in terms of the medical system. Doing this, I can reach a grotesque situation where I tend to forfeit the possibility to live my own life; I can even become little more than an adjunct of the personnel and machines, the dreams and therapies, of medical entrepreneurship."

"But," concludes Hoinacki, citing conversations with Illich, "to be human means to be wary of systems." Ordinary persons, and especially poor and rural people, often know this; they live in natural systems and have not been able to afford artificial systems. People who have never lived without biohealth cannot imagine life without it; people who have experienced some remnants of a natural engagement with *shalom* health are wary of the system of biohealth. But being wary does not keep the system away. It moves in relentlessly like the incoming tide—and occasionally, as with AIDS care in Africa, moves in suddenly like a tidal wave.

So what can we do, those of us who are wary?

It is a very difficult question. Biohealth is ubiquitous in the North, where most of you who are reading this book are from. Biomedicine is ubiquitous worldwide, and biohealth is rapidly following. We cannot stop it, any more than we can stop the tide from coming in. But it gets more difficult: we may not *want* to stop biomedicine, as it has so much to offer with its techniques that work. Yet biohealth now proclaims itself as the natural successor to biomedicine—and its sole distributor. If we cannot turn back the tide of biohealth, is it at least possible to separate it from biomedicine?

Perhaps a story from the Bible will illustrate.[5] During Jesus' time on earth, he found himself involved, sometimes entangled, in two systems: the political system of Rome, under Tiberius Caesar, and the religious system of the Jews, of which the Pharisees were prominent spokesmen. Jesus was wary of these two systems, enough so that supporters of both often tried to get him to show his hand so they would have grounds to arrest him. On one occasion representatives of both came together to ask him if it was permissible to pay taxes, presumably a test of ultimate loyalty.

---

5. Matt 22:15–22.

Jesus' response, I think, gets to the heart of the systems problem, and provides an introduction to our response to biohealth. He took a coin and asked whose image was on it. The answer, Caesar's, was the answer to the dilemma of taxes. *All* money is Caesar's (part of the political system) anyway; paying taxes is just giving it back. But that isn't the end. There is another reality (God) which the Pharisees had tried to hijack with their religious system. That reality, according to Jesus, is what requires our ultimate allegiance.

It is a clever response. Instead of rejecting outright the oppressive political system, Jesus recognized its reality, gave it back what it had produced, then turned his attention to the more important things. It is possible to pay taxes, Jesus was saying, without ultimate loyalty to Caesar. Might this story give us a pattern to respond to biohealth? Might it be possible to use some of the tools of biomedicine without embracing the whole system of biohealth? In this final section, we will return to each of the four main characteristics of biohealth from Part II, looking for examples of biomedical tools we can use outside the authority of biohealth.

SYSTEMS

"Illich says that tools can be used to one's own purposes and systems make a person conform to their purposes."[6] We humans can, in other words, use and control tools, or we can *be* tools, used and controlled by a system. We can use some of the technologies of biomedicine, and intentionally not use others, depending on how those tools enhance our *shalom* health. But when we enter the system of biohealth, and are presented with a package of tools to enable us to fulfill our optimal life trajectory, we in fact become a tool of that trajectory.

The first point is to recognize when what is being offered us is a system. Consider this example: *Vaccination* is a tool, and many vaccinations make sense to me as person who is also a doctor. I keep my tetanus vaccination up to date, and get rabies boosters when I work in communities where there are rabid animals. *Immunization guidelines* developed by professional bodies are part of a system; today these guidelines include vaccinating all children for chicken pox, and all pre-adolescent girls (but not boys!) for HPV (human papilloma virus, a sexually trans-

6. Arney, "Criticizing Institutions."

mitted virus implicated in cervical cancer). Now all these vaccine tools "work," but the vaccine system involves vaccinating all children for over a dozen diseases, involving at least five visits before starting school, and several more after starting. And the diseases range from lethal to trivial, and from common to very rare. But the *system* makes no allowance for these differences, nor for the cost, nor for the sense of dependence on itself that this many vaccinations inculcates.

There is a parallel story with plastic surgery. The ability to remodel body parts surgically is a tool; those with congenital defects or injuries benefit from this tool. But the conceptions and importance of physical beauty are part of the system of media and culture that offers, through biohealth, relief from being ugly—as they define it. Again, it is not the tool that we need be wary of as much as the system that delivers it. We could develop similar arguments for the tools that assist in childbirth— and even, as we shall see, for preventive medicines and screening tests.

RISK

As we have seen, risk thinking has been a foundation of much of biohealth, especially screening and surveillance medicine, as well as the judgments of evidence based medicine (EBM). And, as with systems, there is a difference between the tools used to calculate risk and their applications in the system of biohealth. The tools only claim to measure probability, and they do it well. They help us make very accurate statements and predictions about populations of people. It is the system of biohealth, not the tools of biostatistics, which insists that probability and risk influence what we do clinically with a single patient. We looked at the problems with this in the chapter on risk.

Screening tests themselves offer a picture similar to what we just looked at with vaccines. Some of the tests—for example, taking the blood pressure of a person who feels fine—are inexpensive, painless, and can very effectively identify people who have dangerous and yet treatable high blood pressure. Each well-accepted screening *tool* has some value, as long as we remember that screening is built on probability and risk, not certainty—and that evidence means "statistically significant," not certain.

However, the *system* of screening, like the entire system of bio-health, lacks candor. Look for example at screening for colon cancer.[7] Most colon cancers, more than 80 percent, develop from polyps, and these polyps occasionally bleed. If a person over fifty checks their stool for occult blood every year, that is an indirect way of finding if there are polyps. If there is blood, that person can be further tested, and if polyps are found they can be removed, therefore reducing their risk of cancer. In fact, when large populations of people are screened for blood in their stools, those populations have fewer colon cancers than groups who were not screened. That is the story that the screening system tells—and it is a true story.

However, that is not the whole story. While most cancers do arise from polyps, most polyps do not become cancers. Almost no small ones, and of the ones larger than ten milimeters, only 10 percent will become cancerous within ten years, and only 25 percent within twenty years. More than this, populations of people who are screened for colon cancer do not show any change in overall death rates compared with those who are not screened, although the screened group does have less colon cancer. It would be just as true to tell people: "Four out of five colon cancers come from polyps, and you might have polyps without knowing it. We can find and remove those polyps. However, if you have three polyps and we remove all of them, there is a high chance that none of them would have turned into cancer, and there is a small chance of complications if we do remove them. Even after we give you a "clean bill of health," there is a one in five chance that you will get colon cancer anyway, not arising from a polyp. And even if you do get screened and we remove all the polyps we find, you won't live any longer."

We can choose to do all of the screening tests that biohealth presents to us, and we will be in a group with better health indices than a group that does not get screened. But we may also be more anxious, as we have seen. We could choose to select a few screening tests for very specific reasons—a close relative had a similar condition, for example—as long as we are aware of the limits and risks of screening itself. Or, we could choose to avoid screening altogether, remembering that "those who are well have no need of a physician, but those who are sick."[8] The point is,

7. Rogers et al., "Lower Gastrointestinal Conditions," 13–14.
8. Matt 9:12.

these are all tools that we can use—or not use. The choice belongs to us, not to the system of biohealth.

COMMODITIES

All of these screening tests and vaccines are commodities, things that are produced by biomedicine and sold by biohealth. So are medicines, whether they are preventive medicines, such as cholesterol lowering drugs, or medicines for treatment of disease, like antibiotics or insulin. We have seen that some of the medicines that are most heavily advertised are medicines that we don't *need* in order to live, medicines that are designed to relieve symptoms or reduce our risk of disease. We could view many of these in the same way that we view screening: the choice is ours.

But what of those medicines that cure disease, like antibiotics? Or that keep a person alive, like insulin for diabetics, or ARVs for people with AIDS? Or all the commodities involved with life-saving surgery? Surely this is one place where the gap between the tools of biomedicine and the system of biohealth is narrow. After all, these are complex commodities that require experts, aren't they?

Yes, these tools require expertise, and biomedicine readily provides it. However, as we saw in the chapter on AIDS in Africa, that expertise easily slips into biohealth, and the distinction between the tool and the system gets blurred. Prevention of AIDS, which began as ABC, and then degenerated to A vs C, has now been almost replaced by VCT. It moved from an emphasis on behavior, to an emphasis on a commodity people could control (condoms), to a commodity biomedicine controlled (testing). The entire process is the movement from community activity to biomedicine to biohealth.

The ARV story is somewhat different. Whenever biomedicine develops a drug that keeps people alive as long as they take it—insulin was the first—it must immediately call in the services of biohealth. These commodities, these tools, require a system of perpetual care. It is very difficult here to render to Caesar, and then go on about our business. Chronic disease is Caesar's business. Biohealth finally has legitimacy—almost. The problem is, biohealth does not know how or when to stop.

There is no stopping until the patient, by death, refuses any more ministrations from biohealth.

But we can refuse before we die. I remember the day my brother-in-law refused. He was forty-nine, and dying from colon cancer—apparently one of the 20 percent not originating in a polyp, and therefore not subject to screening. He had chosen initially to use the tools of biomedicine in some of Boston's best hospitals: he had surgery, then chemotherapy. Then another cancer developed: more surgery. Then it spread to his spine and his brain: more chemotherapy, more surgery. Finally it was clear that the tools of biomedicine were exhausted, and he went home (still mobile, still talking, still hurting), this time a patient of Hospice.

We were sitting on his back deck, having supper with our family and his family; it was a pleasant New England summer evening. My sister presented him with the pills he was supposed to be taking. Now Dick was generally a very quiet fellow, not boisterous, not the center of attention. My sister nudged the pills a bit closer. Then Dick picked up one in each hand, and without saying a word, threw them both over the table and into the yard. It wasn't a throw of anger; it was, if anything, a declaration of independence from biohealth.

Those who have chronic diseases, or care for those who do, can feel horribly trapped, especially near the end. There is always another commodity, another tool of biomedicine that biohealth is willing to put before them. There is the financial and physical burden of going on if they take what is offered, and gut-wrenching guilt if they don't. Yet biohealth cannot back off. All it has to offer are commodities, and death is the ultimate sign of its failure. But people know, long before biohealth does, when the end is near. It is up to us to throw our pills into the yard.

RESPONSIBILITY

Biohealth provides us with all sorts of commodities, both to treat disease and increasingly to find it early and treat it before we know we have it. It is also part of a larger technological system that provides us with an overabundance of commodities—not all of which, as we have seen, enhance health. Biohealth then turns around and tells us that health is our responsibility, and that to maintain good health it is up to us to use all of its offerings and avoid all those commodities that damage health.

This is clever reasoning, and most of us fall for it. But there is a flaw: the health that we're told is our responsibility is biohealth, not *shalom* health. Biohealth defines health statistically: we are healthier if our numbers are better and our risks are lower. Using the good commodities of biohealth, and avoiding the bad commodities that damage health, we can get better numbers and lower risk. And it certainly seems up to us to avoid Knowles's "sloth, gluttony, alcoholic intemperance, reckless driving, sexual frenzy and smoking"—assuming they are at the root of poor health.

But *shalom* health is closer to the African concept of health we saw in the last chapter; it has more to do with balance, with being part of a healthy community, with a spiritual conception of the universe, and is never merely physical or biological. That sort of *whole* health cannot be one person's responsibility. How much does gluttony come from irresponsibility, and how much from excessive cheap readily available processed food? How much of pathological smoking has been from personal irresponsibility, and how much from irresponsible manufacture and advertising of cigarettes? Damfo, the healer in Armah's novel *The Healers* is clear: "Healing is work, not gambling. It is the work of inspiration, not manipulation. If we the healers are to do the work of helping to bring our people together again, we need to know such work is the work of a community. It cannot be done by any individual. It should not depend on any single person however heroic he may be. And it can't be done by people who don't understand the healing vocation—no matter how good such people may be as individuals."[9]

To say it differently, individual responsibility for health belongs squarely in the system of biohealth. Biohealth tries to heal individuals without healing communities—a never-ending work because it never touches the root causes of ill health. In fact most of the tools of biomedicine do no better at getting to these roots. Like chronic disease, the biohealth mantra of responsibility belongs to Caesar—and it's OK to pay Caesar tax. But we should never think that we are finished after we have rendered to Caesar what is Caesar's. That only gets Caesar off our backs, and clears the way for us to begin to address the real business of healing.

9. Armah, *Healers*, 308.

These are just a few illustrative examples; biomedicine is loaded with tools we can use in the process of healing. However, we must be clear about what we are proposing in this conclusion. As we look for these tools of biomedicine we can use outside of the authority of biohealth, I am not proposing a way to change the system of biohealth to reduce its influence or mitigate its power. That is impossible. If biohealth—or any technology—truly does come in like a tide, a sensible response can only be to live with the rising water, not try to chase it away. When Caesar rushes in demanding tax, we could refuse—and end up incarcerated. Or we could pay the tax—but we should expect from that tax only biohealth, not *shalom* health.

Yet every technology not only believes itself good and necessary, it believes that any problems that develop can be solved by itself or another technology. Contemporary social critics are caught in the same belief; a template title for many books of social, economic, or political analysis today is *The Problem with X and What to Do About It*. We do not let ourselves believe that our problems are unsolvable. But complex systems such as biohealth cannot be fixed: they are "relentlessly resilient to change, rapidly responsive to criticism, and remarkably stable for it." They are like a bicycle—"self-righting, equilibrium-maintaining"—and they "sustain themselves in response to most assaults from their environments or injuries to their internal workings." Yet when change comes, it unfortunately is also like the bicycle that encounters the unexpected pebble in just the wrong (or right) place in the road: the collapse tends to be catastrophic.[10] Tinkering doesn't help, and catastrophic collapse hurts everyone.

There comes a time when we simply have to say "No." There is the "No" of the activist, a "no" whose refusal is a first step, a clearing away of something to allow for an alternative preplanned "yes." The "No" of the activist creates a hole that needs to be filled—and so it is an optimistic "No," one preparing for the "... and What to Do About It" of the book title. The activist "No" is sure of itself, sometimes impatient and angry; a "No" that cries out and shouts aloud, whose voice is heard in the streets; a "No" that can easily break the bruised reed and quench the wavering flame.

---

10. Arney, *Experts in the Age of Systems*, 5.

There is another "No," the "No" of Herman Melville's "Bartleby the Scrivener."[11] Bartleby was a copyist in a lawyer's office on Wall Street. His two colleagues responded to this tedious meaningless work in very understandable ways: indigestion, carelessness, drinking, losing their tempers—but they both kept on copying and proofreading. Bartleby at first worked very diligently and without complaint—and then one day said simply "I would prefer not to." This was not a strike, not a demand for better working conditions, not a political statement. Bartleby offered no reason for his "No"—or rather his "preference"—and certainly offered no plan. He simply stopped working, but (Melville says in italics) "*he was always there*"; he did not resign. His employer and colleagues were confronted every day with his strange yet very sane "preference."

Bartleby's world was grim; refusing to copy and proofread left him no other options, and he remained idle. What is the lesson for those confronted with biohealth? Biohealth, as we have emphasized throughout this book, is not the same as biomedicine; preferring not to engage with biohealth does not imply repudiating biomedicine. We have, as we saw above, choices. And so, with gratitude to Bartleby:

I would prefer not to be part of the system that tries to manage my life.

I would prefer not to employ risk to determine what I do to be healthy.

I would prefer not to use commodities to maintain health.

I would prefer not to accept responsibility for my biohealth.

Jacques Ellul must have been taken to task for his constant criticism of technological systems without a clear plan about how to fix them. His response at the end of one of his books was a metaphor: A person is bound fast, wrist and ankles, with a well-forged new chain, and I break the chain with a sledgehammer. I can be criticized for this purely negative act—making useless a fine product of human technique, and constructing nothing useful in its place. Yet that "destructive" act is all that is necessary to liberate the person. There is no need for a school to teach unfettered people how to walk—"and if he prefers to stay hunched up in his prison wishing for his chains back, what further positive deed can I do for him?"[12]

---

11. Melville, "Bartleby the Scrivener."
12. Ellul, *Humiliation of the Word*. 268.

In this book I am only trying to make clear the difference between the tools of biomedicine and the system of biohealth, and to give a few examples of tools that are worth prying loose from the system they have become embedded in. The work of healing in this environment is still very difficult, as Damfo says in the quote from *The Healers* above—more difficult than walking after chains have been broken. But we cannot begin until we recognize the chains of biohealth.

Chronology

1848   Hand-washing prevents puerperal fever—Semmelweiss
        General anesthesia for childbirth—Channing

1898   Cause of malaria determined—Ross

1900   ICD (International Classification of Diseases) founded

1901   Electrocardiograph developed
        First Nobel Prize in Medicine—von Behring (antitoxin for
        diphtheria)

1910   Flexner Report

1915   All childbirth "pathological", requires forceps and
        anesthesia—DeLee

1916   First birth control clinic in US—Margaret Sanger

1918   *Married Love*—Marie Stopes

1919   Alcohol Prohibition begun in the US

1921   Insulin isolated—Banting and Best

1923   Diphtheria vaccine developed

1926   Pertussis vaccine developed

1927   Iron lung developed
        Tetanus toxoid developed

1928   Penicillin discovered—Fleming

      Papanicolaou's first work on cytology screening in a eugenics journal

1933   US Prohibition repealed

1935   Blood banks initiated

      Alcoholics Anonymous (AA) begins

1938   First artificial hip implanted

1941   Pap smear developed—George Papanicolaou

1942   DPT combine vaccine available

1940s   Chemotherapy for cancer available

1953   Structure of DNA described—Watson and Crick

1950s   Heart-lung bypass machine

1956   AMA declares alcoholism an illness

1960   Renal dialysis

1960s   Heart, liver, kidney transplantations
      Intensive Care Units
      Community Cardio-Pulmonary Resuscitation (CPR)
      Mammography becomes widespread

1968   ADHD appeared in DSM-II as "hyperkinetic reaction of childhood"
      Social Phobia appeared in DSM-II as "social fears"

1973   Roe v Wade: abortion legalized in the US

1974   Canadian Lalonde Reports launching health promotion

1976   *Medical Nemesis*—Ivan Illich
      Karen Quinlin legal battle for discontinuing ventilator

1977   Biopsychosocial model proposed—Engel

"The Responsibility of the Individual"—Knowles

1978 UN Conference on Primary Health Care—Alma Ata

1979 *The Postmodern Condition*—Lyotard

1980 PSA test introduced for screening for prostate cancer
Ronald Regan elected US president
"The New Medical-Industrial Complex"—Relman

1981 First PC—personal computer
First direct-to-consumer advert of a prescription drug—
Reader's Digest
AIDS first described.

1982 US Supreme Court declares AMA cannot prohibit advertising

1984 *Medicine and the Management of Living*—Arney and Bergen

1986 *Risk Society* published in Germany—Beck

1980s Chronic Fatigue Syndrome described
Just Say No campaign—Nancy Reagan

1997 Direct-to-consumer TV ads begin in US after FDA guidlines

2000 *To Err Is Human*—documenting medical errors
Cosmetic procedures begin to outnumber reconstructive
procedures
Mbeki attempts to articulate an African paradigm to confront
AIDS

2004 US "Future of Family Medicine" New Model

Bibliography

About.com. "The History of Computers." Online: http://inventors.about.com/library/blcoindex.htm.

———. "Social Anxiety Disorder: A Brief History of the Disorder." Online: http://socialanxietydisorder.about.com/od/overviewofsad/a/history.htm

Achebe, C., G. Hyden, C. Magadza, and A. P. Okeyo. *Beyond Hunger in Africa: Conventional Wisdom and an African Vision*. Nairobi: Heinemann Kenya, 1990.

American Society of Plastic Surgeons. "Media—Statistics." Online: http://www.plasticsurgery.org.

Ameringer, Carl. "Organized Medicine on Trial: The Federal Trade Commission vs. the American Medical Association." *Journal of Policy History* 12 (2000) 445–71.

Angell, Marcia. *The Truth About the Drug Companies: How They Deceive Us and What To Do About It*. New York: Random House, 2004.

Armah, Ayi Kwei. *The Healers: A Novel*. Popenguine, Senegal: Per Ankh, 2000.

Armstrong, David. "The Rise of Surveillance Medicine." *Sociology of Health & Illness* 17 (1995) 393–404.

———. "Use of the Genealogical Method in the Exploration of Chronic Illness: A Research Note." *Soc. Sci. Med.* 30 (1990) 1225–27.

Arney, William Ray. "Criticizing Institutions in the Age of Systems? Might as Well Criticize Life." Unpublished paper given at a colloquium called "Conviviality in the Age of Systems," Cuernavaca, Mexico, December, 2007.

———. *Experts in the Age of Systems*. Albuquerque: University of New Mexico Press, 1991.

Arney, William Ray, and B. Bergen. *Medicine and the Management of Living: Taming the Last Great Beast*. Chicago: University of Chicago Press, 1984.

Babes, A. "Diagnostic du cancer du col uterin par les frottes." *Presse Med* 36 (1927) 451.

Backstein, R., and A. Hinek. "War and Medicine: The Origins of Plastic Surgery." *University of Toronto Medical Journal* 82 (2005) 217–19.

Bacon, Francis. *New Atlantis*. In *Three Early Modern Utopias*, edited by Susan Bruce Oxford: Oxford University Press, 1999.

Baldwin Research Institute. "Alcoholism: A Disease of Speculation." Online: http://www.baldwinresearch.com/alcoholism.cfm.

Bálint G. P., W. F. Kean, and W. W. Buchanan. "Sir William Osler (1849–1919) His Opinion of Modern Therapeutics." *Scottish Medical Journal* 50 (2006) 51–53.

Barasky, A. "The Paradox of Health." *NEJM* 318 (1988) 414–18.

Beck, Ulrich. *Risk Society: Towards a New Modernity.* London: Sage, 1992.

Berlinguer, G. "Bioethics, Health, and Inequality." *Lancet* 364 (2004) 1086–91.

Blumenthal J., et al. "Effects of Exercise Training on Older Patients with Major Depression." *Arch Intern Med* 159 (1999) 2349–56.

BrainyQuote—William Osler. No pages. Online: http://www.brainyquote.com/quotes/authors/w/william_osler.html

Bujo, Benezet. *The Ethical Dimension of Community: The African Model and the Dialogue Between North and South.* Nairobi: Paulines, 1998.

Centers for Disease Control and Prevention (CDC). Online: http://www.cdc.gov/mmwr/preview/mmwrhtml/00056803.html.

Chesterton, G. K. *Eugenics and Other Evils: An Argument Against the Scientifically Organized State.* Seattle, WA: Inkling, 2000.

Claiborne, Robert. *The Roots of English.* New York: Anchor, 1989.

Clarke, Shim, et al. "Biomedicalization: Technoscientific Transformations of Health, Illness, and U.S. Biomedicine." *American Sociological Review* 68 (2003) 161–94.

Clarke, A. E. "From the Rise of Medicine To Biomedicalization: U.S. Healthscapes and Iconography c1890-Present, With Global Implications." Speech given to the 2nd EASTS Conference, August 6–8, 2007. Handout Online: http://stsweb.ym.edu.tw/easts/2007/clarke.pdf.

Conrad, Peter. "The Shifting Engines of Medicalization." *Journal of Health and Social Behaviour* 46 (2005) 3–14.

Crawford, Robert. "Health as a Meaningful Social Practice." *Health: An Interdisciplinary Journal for the Social Study of Health, Illness, and Medicine* 10 (2006) 401–20.

———. "Risk Ritual and the Management of Control and Anxiety in Medical Culture." *Health: An Interdisciplinary Journal for the Social Study of Health, Illness, and Medicine* 8 (2004) 505–28.

D'Adesky, Anne-Christine. *Moving Mountains: The Race to Treat Global AIDS.* London: Verso, 2004.

Declaration of Alma-Ata, 1978. Online: http://www.who.int/hpr/NPH/docs/declaration_almaata.pdf.

Donohue, J., et al. "A Decade of Direct-to-Consumer Advertising of Prescription Drugs." *NEJM* 357 (2007) 673–81.

Downing, Raymond. *As They See It: The Development of the African AIDS Discourse.* London: Adonis & Abbey, 2005.

———. *Death and Life in America: A Dialogue Between Biblical Healing and Biomedicine.* Scottdale, PA: Herald, 2008.

———. *Suffering and Healing in America: An American Doctor's View From Outside.* Oxford: Radcliffe, 2006.

———. *The Wedding Goes On Without Us.* Nairobi: Jacaranda Designs, 2001.

Dubos, René. *Mirage of Health: Utopias, Progress, and Biological Change.* New York: Harper & Row, 1959.

Duden, Barbara. *Disembodying Women: Perspectives on Pregnancy and the Unborn* Cambridge: Harvard University Press, 1993.

———. "Ivan Illich. Beyond Medical Nemesis (1976) The Search for Modernity's Disembodiment of 'I' and 'You.'" Notes for a symposium, February 7–8, 2003. Online: http://www.pudel.uni-bremen.de/pdf/Iv_tra_b.pdf, 5–6.

———. "The Quest for Past Somatics." In *The Challenges of Ivan Illich: A Collective Reflection*, edited by Lee Hoinacki and Carl Mitcham, 219–30. Albany: State University of New York Press, 2002.

Durst, Dennis. "Evangelical Engagements with Eugenics 1900–1940." *Ethics & Medicine* 18 (2002). Online: http://findarticles.com/p/articles/mi_qa4004/is_200207/ai_n9119561/.

Ebell, Mark. "Information Mastery." FP Essentials No. 318, AAFP Home Study. Leawood, KA: American Academy of Family Physicians, 2006.

Editorial. "Margaret Chan Puts Primary Health Care Centre Stage at WHO." *The Lancet* 371 (2008) 1811.

Ehrenreich, John. "Introduction: The Cultural Crisis of Modern Medicine." In *The Cultural Crisis of Modern Medicine*, edited by John Ehrenreich, 1–35. New York: Monthly Review, 1978.

Eli Lilly. "ADHD Timeline." 2008. Online: www.lilly.com/news/pdf/RG_ADHD_time_00000012.pdf.

Elliot, Carl. *Better Than Well: American Medicine Meets the American Dream*. New York: Norton, 2003.

Ellul, Jacques. *The Humiliation of the Word*. Grand Rapids: Eerdmans, 1985.

———. *Propaganda: The Formation of Men's Attitudes*. New York: Vintage, 1973.

———. *The Technological Society*. New York: Vintage, 1964.

———. *The Technological System*. New York: Continuum, 1980.

Engel, George. "The Need for a New Medical Model: A Challenge for Biomedicine." *Science* 196 (1977) 129–36.

Fanon, Franz. "Medicine and Colonialism." In *The Cultural Crisis of Modern Medicine*, edited by John Ehrenreich, 229–51. New York: Monthly Review, 1978.

FDA website. Online: http://www.fda.gov/AboutFDA/WhatWeDo/History/Product Regulation/SummaryofNDAApprovalsReceipts1938tothepresent/default.htm.

Feldhusen, Adrian. "The History of Midwifery and Childbirth in America: A Timeline." Online: http://www.midwiferytoday.com/articles/timeline.asp.

File, D. "The Medical Text: Between Biomedicine and Hegemony." *Social Science and Medicine* 59 (2004) 1275–85.

Filion, Yves. "The Moral Impotence of Contemporary Experts." *Bulletin of Science, Technology, & Society* 24 (2004) 342–52.

Fox, Daniel. *Power and Illness: The Failure and Future of American Health Policy*. Berkeley: University of California Press, 1993.

Galvin, Rose. "Disturbing Notions of Chronic Illness and Individual Responsibility: Towards a Genealogy of Morals." *Health* 6 (2002) 107–37.

George Papanicolaou. Essortment Web site. Online: http://www.essortment.com/uterinecancerp_ruxf.html.

Giddens, Anthony. *Runaway World: How Globalisation is Reshaping our Lives*. London: Profile, 2002.

Gisselquist, D. "Denialism Undermines AIDS Prevention in Sub-Saharan Africa." *International Journal of STD & AIDS* 19 (2008) 649–55.

Graham, Linda. "The Politics of ADHD." *Proceedings Australian Association for Research in Education (AARE) Annual Conference 2006*. Online: http://www.aare.edu.au/06pap/gra06090.pdf.

Green L., et al. "Task Force 1. Report of the Task Force on Patient Expectations, Core Values, Reintegration, and the New Model of Family Medicine." *Annals of Family Medicine* 2 (2004) S33–S50.

Green, Edward. *Rethinking AIDS Prevention: Learning from Successes in Developing Countries.* Westport, CT: Praeger, 2003.

Gross, L. S., et al. "Increased consumption of refined carbohydrates and the epidemic of type 2 diabetes in the United States: an ecologic assessment." *American Journal of Clinical Nutrition* 79 (2004) 774–79.

Gutierrez, C., and P. Scheid, "The History of Family Medicine and Its Impact in US Health Care Delivery." Paper presented at the Primary Care Symposium at the University of California, San Diego, May 29, 2002. Online: http://www.aafpfoundation.org/PreBuilt/foundation_gutierrezpaper.pdf.

Hadler, Nortin. *The Last Well Person: How to Stay Well Despite the Health-Care System.* Montreal: McGill-Queen's University Press, 2004.

Haiken, Elizabeth. *Venus Envy: A History of Cosmetic Surgery.* Baltimore: Johns Hopkins University Press, 1997.

Hall, Amy Laura. *Conceiving Parenthood: American Protestantism and the Spirit of Reproduction.* Grand Rapids: Eerdmans, 2008.

Hall, W. "Biomedicalization of Alcohol Studies: Ideological Shifts and Institutional Challenges." *Addiction* 102 (2007) 494–95.

Hoinacki, Lee. *Dying Is Not Death.* Eugene, OR: Wipf & Stock, 2006.

Illich, Ivan. "Brave New Biocracy: Health Care from Womb to Tomb." *New Perspectives Quarterly* 11:1 (1994). Online: http://www.davidtinapple.com/illich/1994_biocracy.html

———. "Heath as One's Own Responsibility—No Thank You!" Speech given September 14, 1990. Online: http://www.davidtinapple.com/illich/1990_health_responsibility.PDF.

———. "Hospitality and Pain." Presented in Chicago in 1987. Online: http://www.davidtinapple.com/illich/1987_hospitality_and_pain.PDF.

———. "Medical Ethics: A Call to De-bunk Bio-ethics." In *In the Mirror of the Past: Lectures and Addresses 1978–1990.* London: Marion Boyars, 1992.

———. *Medical Nemesis: The Expropriation of Health.* New York: Pantheon, 1976.

———. "Pathogenesis, Immunity, and the Quality of Public Health." *Qualitative Health Research* 5:1 (1995). Online: http://academic.evergreen.edu/curricular/hhd2000/Rita/PATHOGENESIS.htm.

———. *The Right to Useful Unemployment and its Professional Enemies.* London: Marion Boyars, 1978.

———. *The Rivers North of the Future.* Toronto: Anansi, 2005.

———. *Tools for Conviviality.* New York: Harper & Row, 1973.

Kanyandago, Peter. "AIDS in Africa: Anthropological and Ethical Questions." Presented at Nkozi, Uganda, August 28–September 1, 2000. Online: www.africanaids.org/media/kanyand.pdf.

Kass, Amalie. "'My Brother Preaches, I Practice': Walter Channing, M.D., Antebellum Obstetrician." *Massachusetts Historical Review.* Online: http://www.historycooperative.org/journals/mhr/1/kass.html.

Katongole, Emmanuel. "An Age of Miraculous Medicines." In *AIDS in Africa: Theological Reflections,* edited by B. Bujo and M. Czerny, 104–19. Nairobi: Paulines, 2007.

Khan, N., et al. "The Future of Family Medicine: A Collaborative Project of the Family Medicine Community." *Annals of Family Medicine* 2 (2004) Supplement 1, S3–S32.

Knowler, W. C., et al. "Reduction in the Incidence of Type 2 Diabetes with Lifestyle Intervention or Metformin." *N Engl J Med* 346 (2002) 393–403.

Koenig, Michael, and Elizabeth Mezick. "Are Pharmaceutical Company Mergers Rational?" *The Scientist* 18 (2004). Online: http://www.vetscite.org/publish/items/001761/index .html.

Kohn L. T., J. Corrigan, and M. S. Donaldson. *To Err Is Human. Building a Safer Health System*. Institute of Medicine. Washington, DC: National Academy, 2000.

Kotlowski, D. J. "The Knowles Affair: Nixon's Self-Inflicted Wound." *Presidential Studies Quarterly* 30 (2000) 443–62.

Kugelmann, Robert. "Health in the Light of a Critical Health Psychology." *Psicologia desde el Caribe. Universidad del Norte* 11 (2003) 75–93.

Lander, Louise. *Defective Medicine: Risk, Anger, and the Malpractice Crisis*. New York: Farrar Straus & Giroux, 1978.

Lantz, P., et al. "Socioeconomic Factors, Health Behaviors, and Mortality." *JAMA* 279 (1998) 1703–8.

Le Fanu, James. *The Rise and Fall of Modern Medicine*. New York: Carroll & Graf, 1999.

Leeder, S. R. "The New Public Health." 2005. Online: http://www.menzieshealthpolicy. edu.au/media/doc/nphtnvlo70305.pdf.

Life Line Screening Pamphlet. Online: http://www.lifelinescreening.com.

Lipworth, L., et al. "Excess Mortality From Suicide and Other External Causes of Death Among Women With Cosmetic Breast Implants." *Annals of Plastic Surgery* 59 (2007) 119–23.

Little, Margaret Olivia. "Cosmetic Surgery, Suspect Norms, and the Ethics of Complicity." In *Enhancing Human Traits: Ethical and Social Implications*, edited by Erik Parens. Washington, DC: Georgetown University Press, 1998.

Loewy, E. "Bioethics: Past, Present, and an Open Future." *Cambridge Quarterly of Healthcare Ethics* 11 (2002) 388–97.

Lyotard, Jean-François. *The Postmodern Condition: A Report on Knowledge*. Online: http://www.idehist.uu.se/distans/ilmh/pm/lyotard-introd.htm.

Magesa, Laurenti. *African Religion: The Moral Traditions of Abundant Life*. Maryknoll, NY: Orbis, 1997.

———. *Christian Ethics in Africa*. Nairobi: Acton, 2002.

Mbeki, Thabo. "Letter to World Leaders." Online: http://www.tinevandermaas.com/ background-info/thabo-mbeki-letter-to-world-leaders/

———. Interview with Debra Patta, April 24, 2001 on eTV "On The Record." Online: http://www.search.gov.za/info/previewDocument.jsp?dk=%2Fdata%2Fstatic%2Fi nfo%2Fspeeches%2F2001%2F010504945a1001.htm%40Gov&q=(+(aids%3CAN D%3Epanel)+)&t=Transcription+of+e.tv+interview+with+President+Thabo+Mb eki.

McKeown, Thomas. *The Role of Medicine: Dream, Mirage, or Nemesis?* Princeton: Princeton University Press, 1979.

Meador, Clifton. "The Last Well Person." *NEJM* 330 (1994) 440–41.

Melville, Herman. "Bartleby the Scrivener, A Tale of Wall Street." Online: http://www. enotes.com/bartleby-scrivener-text.

Mendelsohn, Robert. *Confessions of a Medical Heretic*. New York: Warner, 1979.

Merchant, Carolyn. *The Death of Nature: Women, Ecology and the Scientific Revolution.* San Francisco: HarperSanFrancisco, 1980.

Meridian Institute. "The Relation of Chronic Fatigue Syndrome and Neurasthenia." Online: http://www.meridianinstitute.com/neurasth.htm.

Merriam-Webster. *Merriam-Webster's Collegiate Dictionary.* Springfield, MA: Merriam Webster, 2004.

Miron, J. A. "Alcohol Prohibition." EH.Net Encyclopedia Web site. Online: http://eh.net/encyclopedia/article/miron.prohibition.alcohol.

Mitcham, C. "Unexpected Friendship." *Whole Earth* 111 (Spring 2003). Online: http://wholeearth.com/issue/111/article/181/remembering.ivan.illich.

Morabia, A., and F. F. Zhang. "History of Medical Screening: From Concepts to Action." *Postgrad Med J* 80 (2004) 463–69.

Mori, M. "The Twilight of 'Medicine' and the Dawn of 'Health Care': Reflections on Bioethics at the Turn of the Millennium." *Journal of Medicine and Philosophy* 25 (2000) 723–44.

Morris, David B. *Illness and Culture in the Postmodern Age.* Berkeley: University of California Press, 1998.

Moynihan, R., I. Health, and D. Henry. "Selling Sickness: The Pharmaceutical Industry and Disease Mongering." *BMJ* 324 (2002) 886–91.

Mudimbe, V. Y. *The Invention of Africa: Gnosis, Philosophy, and the Order of Knowledge.* Bloomington: Indiana University Press, 1988.

Nestle, Marion. *Food Politics: How the Food Industry Influences Nutrition and Health.* Berkeley: University of California Press, 2002.

Nye, Robert. "The Evolution of the Concept of Medicalization in the Late Twentieth Century." *Journal of History of the Behavioral Sciences* 39 (2003) 115–29.

O'Malley, K. J., et al. "Measuring Diagnoses: ICD Code Accuracy." *Health Services Research* 40 (2005) 1620–39.

O'Rourke, K. "As Time Goes By: Twenty-Five Years of Bioethics." *Cambridge Quarterly of Healthcare Ethics* 11 (2002) 380–87.

Packard, Vance. *The Hidden Persuaders.* New York: David McKay, 1957.

Papanicolaou, G. N. "New Cancer Diagnosis." In *Proceedings of the Third Race Betterment Conference.* Battle Creek, MI: Race Betterment Foundation 1928.

Papanicolaou, G. N., and H. Traut. "The Diagnostic Value of Vaginal Smears in Carcinoma of the Uterus." *American Journal of Obstetrics and Gynecology* 42 (1941) 193–206.

Payer, Lynn. *Medicine and Culture: Varieties of Treatment in the United States, England, West Germany, and France.* New York: Henry Holt, 1988.

Peterson, A., and D. Lupton. *The New Public Health: Health and Self in the Age of Risk.* London: Sage, 1996.

Pierce, M., et al. "More Good than Harm: A Randomised Controlled Trial of the Effect of Education about Familial Risk of Diabetes on Psychological Outcomes." *Br J Gen Pract* 50 (2000) 867–71.

Public Citizen Congress Watch. "2002 Drug Industry Profits" (2003) 12. Online: http://www.citizen.org/documents/Pharma_Report.pdf

Reiser, Stanley Joel. *Medicine and the Reign of Technology.* Cambridge: Cambridge University Press, 1978.

Relman, Arnold. "The Future of Medical Practice." 1982. Online: http://content.healthaffairs.org/cgi/reprint/2/2/5.pdf.

————. "The New Medical-Industrial Complex." *NEJM* 303 (1980) 963–70.

Rempel, Henry. *A High Price for Abundant Living: The Story of Capitalism.* Waterloo, Ontario: Herald, 2003.

Ridzon, R., et al. "Simultaneous Transmission of Human Immunodeficiency Virus and Hepatitis C Virus from a Needle-Stick Injury." *NEJM* 336 (1997) 919–22.

Roe v Wade. 1973. Online: http://www.tourolaw.edu/Patch/Roe/.

Rogers, J. C., et al. "Lower Gastrointestinal Conditions." *FP Essentials.* Edition No. 345, AAFP Home Study, Leawood, Kansas, February, 2008.

Rooks, Judith. "Childbirth: The History of Childbearing Choices in the United States." Online: http://www.ourbodiesourselves.org/book/companion.asp?id=22&comp ID=75.

Rose, Nikolas. "Beyond Medicalisation." *Lancet* 396 (2007) 700–702.

————. "Molecular Biopolitics, Somatic Ethics and the Spirit of Biocapital." *Social Theory and Health* 5 (2007) 3–29.

————. "The Politics of Life Itself." *Theory, Culture, and Society* 18 (2001) 1–30.

Rosen, George. *A History of Public Health.* Baltimore: Johns Hopkins University Press, 1993.

Rosenthal M., et al. "Promotion of Prescription Drugs to Consumers." *NEJM* 346 (2002) 498–505.

Scherger, J. "The End of the Beginning: The Redesign Imperative in Family Medicine." *Family Medicine* 37 (2005) 513–16.

Schneider, J. W. "Deviant Drinking as Disease: Alcoholism as a Social Accomplishment." *Social Problems* 25 (1978) 361–72.

Scott, S., and R. Freeman. "Prevention as a Problem of Modernity: The Example of HIV and AIDS." In *Medicine, Health and Risk: Sociological Approaches,* edited by Jonathan Gabe, 151–70. Oxford: Blackwell, 1995.

Seri, Istvan. "Historical Perspectives: Perinatal Profiles: Childbed Fever and Ignác Fülöp Semmelweis." *NeoReviews* 8 (2007) e235–e238. Online: http://neoreviews. aappublications.org/cgi/content/full/neoreviews;8/6/e235.

Starfield, Barbara. "Is US Health Really the Best in the World?" *JAMA* 284 (2000) 483–85.

Starr, Paul. *The Social Transformation of American Medicine.* New York: Basic, 1982.

Steinberg, Jonny. "Not a Disease You Look For." *The Guardian Weekly,* January 23, 2009, 25–27.

Stevens, Rosemary. "The Americanization of Family Medicine: Contradictions, Challenges, and Change, 1969–2000." *Family Medicine* 33 (2001) 232–43.

Stewart-Brown, S., and A. Farmer. "Screening Could Seriously Damage your Health." *BMJ* 314 (1997) 533.

Stivers, Richard. *Technology as Magic: The Triumph of the Irrational.* New York: Continuum, 1999.

Stoate, H. G. "Can Health Screening Damage your Health?" *Journal of the Royal College of General Practitioners* 39 (1989) 193–95.

Szasz, Thomas. *The Theology of Medicine.* Syracuse, NY: Syracuse University Press, 1977.

Tackla, Michelle. "Phoenix from the Flames," "Cultural Shifts and Rifts," and "Cultural Turn, Turn, Turn" in *Cosmetic Surgery Time,* October 1, 2003, November 1, 2003, and January 1, 2004.

Tesh, S. N. *Hidden Arguments: Political Ideology and Disease Prevention Policy* New Brunswick, NJ: Rutgers University Press, 1988.

Thomasma, D. "Early Bioethics." *Cambridge Quarterly of Healthcare Ethics* 11 (2002) 5–6.

Tomycz, N. D. "A Profession Selling Out: Lamenting the Paradigm Shift in Physician Advertising." *J Med Ethics* 32 (2006) 26–28.

Toulmin, S. "How Medicine Saved the Life of Ethics." *Perspectives in Biology and Medicine* 25 (1982) 736–50.

University of Toronto Library Web site. The Discovery and Early Development of Insulin. Online: http://link.library.utoronto.ca/insulin/index.html.

US Department of Health and Human Services. USPSTF Web site. Online: http://www.ahrq.gov/clinic/uspstfix.htm.

White, W. "Addiction as a Disease: Birth of a Concept." *Counselor* 1 (2000) 46–51, 73.

———. "The Rebirth of the Disease Concept of Alcoholism in the 20th Century." *Counselor* 1 (2000) 62–66.

Wilkinson, Richard. *Unhealthy Societies: The Afflictions of Inequality.* London: Routledge, 1996.

Woloshin, S., et al. "Direct-to-Consumer Advertisements for Prescription Drugs: What are Americans Being Sold?" *The Lancet* 358 (2001) 1141–46.

World Health Organization. WHO Statistical Information System. Online: http://www.who.int/whosis/data/Search.jsp?indicators=[Indicator].[MBD].Members.

Yach, D., et al. "Epidemiologic and Economic Consequences of the Global Epidemics of Obesity and Diabetes." *Nature Medicine* 12 (2006) 65.

Yamada, S., and N. Palafox. "On the Biopsychosocial Model: The Example of Political Economic Causes of Diabetes in the Marshall Islands." *Fam Med* 33 (2001) 702–4.

Zola, Irving Kenneth. "Healthism and Disabling Medicalization." In *Disabling Professions*, edited by Ivan Illich. London: Marion Boyars, 1977.

———. "Medicine as an Institution of Social Control." *Sociological Review* 20 (1972) 487–504.

Index

www.ingramcontent.com/pod-product-compliance
Lightning Source LLC
Chambersburg PA
CBHW061738270326
41928CB00011B/2280